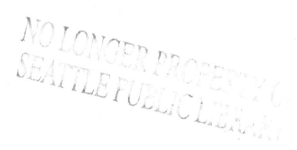

The End of Old Age

The End of Old Age

Living a Longer, More Purposeful Life

Marc E. Agronin, MD

Da Capo

LIFE LONG

Da Capo Press
Hachette Book Group
1290 Avenue of the Americas, New York, NY 10104
www.dacapopress.com
@DaCapoPress; @DaCapoPR

Printed in the United States of America

First Edition: January 2018

Published by Da Capo Lifelong Books, an imprint of Perseus Books, LLC, a subsidiary of Hachette Book Group, Inc. The Da Capo Lifelong Books name and logo is a trademark of the Hachette Book Group.

The Hachette Speakers Bureau provides a wide range of authors for speaking events. To find out more, go to www.hachettespeakersbureau.com or call (866) 376-6591.

The publisher is not responsible for websites (or their content) that are not owned by the publisher.

Library of Congress Cataloging-in-Publication Data
Names: Agronin, Marc E., author.
Title: The end of old age : living a longer, more purposeful life / Marc E. Agronin.
Description: First edition. | New York, NY : Da Capo, 2018 | Includes bibliographical references.
Identifiers: LCCN 2017037867| ISBN 9780738219981 (hardcover) | ISBN 9780738219998 (ebook)
Subjects: | MESH: Aging | Aged | Quality of Life | Health Knowledge, Attitudes, Practice | Popular Works
Classification: LCC QP86 | NLM WT 120 | DDC 612.6/7—dc23
LC record available at https://lccn.loc.gov/2017037867

ISBNs: 978-0-7382-1998-1 (hardcover); 978-0-7382-1999-8 (ebook)

10 9 8 7 6 5 4 3 2 1

Contents

A Note from the Author

*Even if I could have done, when I was young, what I am doing
now—I wouldn't have dared.*

—HENRI MATISSE

THIS BOOK HAS a simple message: *aging brings strength*. When
we realize the truth of this message, we can begin to end the tired
and constricted notions of "old" that we internalize throughout
our lifetime and that serve to denigrate and limit our aging self
and perpetuate an ageist culture. To achieve this understanding,
we must recognize the immense potential of our aging self, even
in the face of common and expected struggles. We must learn how
to age in a creative manner that is both the antidote to feeling old
and the elixir of aging well.

In writing this book, however, I have been confronted with the
absence of certain terms to capture many of the ideas and themes
to support this message. There is a whole language to talk about
growth and development from childhood to adulthood, but for
old age we find an undefined plain that is further obscured by

pejorative labels. I have found it necessary, then, to redefine several key terms and create new ones about aging, to advance my arguments. I am not so bold as to suggest that these terms could or should be part of a larger discussion beyond the confines of this book, but I do welcome a new way of talking about aging that will echo and support these positive points.

Most of the individuals whom I interviewed and feature throughout the book gave me permission to use their actual names, and were eager to share their life histories with me and with readers. In several circumstances, I have changed the name or other identifying biographical details so as to preserve anonymity, especially for individuals who passed away long before I began writing their stories. My goal is to learn about aging from each of these generous individuals, and to both share and celebrate in these pages all the wisdom they have gained throughout their lives.

The seeds of this book began on a shaded porch just outside Washington, DC, in late summer of 2010, when I had the distinct life-changing honor to spend a few hours with Dr. Gene Cohen to talk about the aging process. Unbeknownst to me at the time, this visionary was in the last few months of his life, and yet he took the time to impart his knowledge and guide my thinking despite the underlying pain and worry that he was facing. The young doctor who walked onto that porch was not the same person who left a few hours later, and I am dedicating this book to Gene's memory in the humble hope that I may continue his legacy and join the ongoing work of his life partner, Wendy Miller, to understand and promote creative aging.

Old Is the Problem and Aging Is the Solution

MOST OF US envision living a very long life, and we wonder and scheme how to get there. Now imagine if I told you that I had discovered several potential secrets to achieve this, and I laid them before you on three covered silver trays. You uncover the first and discover a small glass bottle containing genuine water from the fabled Fountain of Youth. You uncover the second tray and discover a pill bottle with a brightly colored label touting a formula designed to add years to your life. Finally, you lift the cover off the third tray and discover, to your surprise, two cigarettes, a glass of red port wine, and several French chocolates.

Which would you choose? You might be bemused by the water and tempted to take a sip, but you realize, no doubt, that it is a gimmick and nothing more. The mysterious supplement in the pill bottle may be bolstered by fantastic claims on its label, but there is no solid proof of its power, and any potential benefit is only a guess. And then there is the strangest choice of all—the smokes, the drink, and the candy. If you choose to indulge in one or more of these treats, you may be guaranteed some brief pleasures—but long life? It seems unlikely. But there is, of course, a story behind this last choice.

Perhaps you have heard of a French woman by the name of Jeanne Louise Calment, the oldest person in recorded human history, who died in 1997 at the age of 122 years and 164 days. As a young girl, she watched the Eiffel Tower being built and later recalled the likes of a rather scruffy and unpleasant artist by the name of Vincent van Gogh who used to frequent her father's fabric store. When she was ninety years old, an enterprising forty-seven-year-old lawyer made an agreement with Madame Calment to pay her a monthly stipend in exchange for her property upon her passing. Unbeknownst to poor Mr. Raffray, however, he would be making payments to this supercentenarian for the next thirty years, up until his own death, after which his widow continued their financial obligation for another two years. When asked about her secret to such a long life, Madame Calment pointed to her lifestyle: she loved regular servings of port wine and chocolate, was physically active but not an exercise fanatic, and smoked two cigarettes daily up to the age of 117. Her longevity strategy, planned or not, certainly seems both unreliable and idiosyncratic, but it is not unlike similarly strange secrets of other supercentenarians.

For example, there was the remarkable Dutch lady Hendrikje van Andel-Schipper. At the age of 112, Hendrikje underwent extensive cognitive testing and scored above average for someone forty years her junior. Her mental clarity remained extraordinary up until the day of her death four years later. An autopsy of her brain revealed few of the telltale pathological signs of similarly aged brains, such as narrowed, sclerotic blood vessels, or plaques containing the toxic amyloid protein associated with Alzheimer's disease. Predictably, Hendrikje was neither teetotaler nor triathlete, and engaged in none of the popular antiaging strategies, such as a vegan diet, caloric restriction, vigorous exercise, or any other youth-restoring pill, potion, or plan. When asked about her secret to a long life, Hendrikje—much like our friend Madame

Calment—revealed a simple and surprising routine: a daily dose of raw herring and a glass of orange juice. The oldest Japanese person ever—117-year-old Misao Okawa—attributed her longevity to sushi and sleep. The Italian 116-year-old Emma Morano cited raw eggs and brandy as her secret formula, whereas the American 116-year-old Susannah Mushatt Jones eschewed alcohol and cigarettes but included at least four strips of bacon in her daily diet.

Do any of these examples mean that we should trash the treadmill and fire up the eggs and bacon? Obviously not. It is clear that none of these supposed secrets to a long life is a reliable strategy, and that some other factors must be at play. Research into the lives of centenarians and the long-lived communities in which many of them reside (the so-called Blue Zones) have all revealed several shared elements of healthy lifestyles, including regular physical activity, close family, or community attachments, and Mediterranean-like diets laden with fish, fruits, vegetables, olive oil, and even a glass of wine. Endless books happily expand upon all these strategies, many plumped with a healthy dose of antiaging sentiment. In the end, however, we know of no surefire strategy or genetic endowment that brings certainty of joining the ranks of these superelders. And we must face a well-recognized truth: a *long* life doesn't necessarily equal a *good* life, and in many circumstances, long in years brings letdowns, languishing, and lots and lots of struggles. Being old, in many ways for many people, seems more of a problem than a promise.

෨

Maybe in our quest for a long life, then, we are missing the point. As a geriatric psychiatrist who has worked for most of my career in the epicenter of aging that is South Florida, I have a unique vantage point to witness the endpoints of these long lives. I get to see whether people actually reap what they sow. And studying aging in Miami is like embarking on a diver's pilgrimage to the Great Blue Hole: a wondrous abyss teeming with old in every hue, form, and layer. I have seen the best and the worst of old age: moneyed and destitute, vibrant and withdrawn, sturdy and decrepit. Sometimes one of these attributes singly defines a person; more often they are all balled up together in a seemingly contradictory but functioning person. In my quest, I have read and researched the vast ocean of thinking, data, musings, and hucksterisms on old age, trying to apprehend and understand the great old white whale into whose mouth I am drawn closer every day. My advantage in writing about aging is not that I am that old myself, but that my life's work has brought the whole beast into my hands. So, let me tell you what I've learned. This is not the old age of times gone by. It's not even the old age that I saw when I began my career in geriatrics some twenty years ago. My average patients are now in their mid- to late eighties and early nineties and, despite lots of daunting medical and psychiatric issues, they are less concerned about living a long life and more focused on living a life full of purpose and meaning. We are so concerned about making our body and brain younger, but perhaps these aged individuals have something special to teach us about the actual strengths of aging that we only gain with time.

My former patient Leah, for example, was a well-known political activist in Miami who began life in a down-and-out Brooklyn borough and spent years thinking that her life was limited to only being a caregiver for her disabled daughter. Aging liberated her activist instincts, however, and in her later years she spent each election cycle fiercely stumping for her favorite candidates, leading get-out-the-vote campaigns in her community, and rallying against the opposing party in newspaper and television interviews. With age, Leah emerged as a more vibrant, opinionated, and dedicated individual whose interests and activism peaked in her nineties and continued unabated until her death at the age of 106. Another example is my patient Eduardo, who used to come for monthly psychotherapy sessions decked out in jeans and designer shirts. In his eighties he continued to grow and diversify the business he had started some fifty years earlier, and in his nineties he continued to mentor two generations of offspring on his work ethic and business acumen. You may argue that Leah and Ed are both exceptions and exceptional, but I am seeing more Leahs and Eduardos every day. Older? Yes. Sicker? In some ways, yes. But scratch the veneer of the typical "old person" that we perceive only through our limited, youthful goggles and a bursting, blooming culture appears of someone engaged in important artistic activities, business transactions, community events, intergenerational relationships, and spiritual endeavors that are rich, varied, life-sustaining, and sometimes jaw-dropping in their intensity and influence. Whether they know it or not, these individuals are plotting the end of old age, a veritable redefining and resculpting of the aging process whereby the narrow and negative paradigm of "old" that we believe in is simply no longer true.

If you want to see the end of this tired notion of old age, then, just open your eyes to the growing legions of relatively healthy and hearty aging individuals who are living, working, playing, and serving vital roles in every one of our communities. For myself, I live in the state of Florida, which has four of the top ten counties in the United States with the highest percentage of individuals older than the age of sixty-five. Here you will find burgeoning retirement communities draping the local interstates like the big fat pomelos hanging off trees in the surrounding citrus groves. You will also find the actual spring of water dubbed the "Fountain of Youth" in a small park in the city of Saint Augustine, where Ponce de León reportedly first set foot on these shores back in 1513. But neither magical waters nor the promise of youth are what these waves of seniors here and elsewhere seek. Their aim is not simply to rest their aching bones for a few happy years before dying—as life after retirement has traditionally been envisioned. Quite the contrary: they intend to live a good life that age itself has granted—in places where age is king and youth is simply in the way. Call it what you will—an *age wave* or *silver tsunami*—but it's hitting big in every developed country, spreading fast and busting with tens of millions of individuals continually adding to its ranks. And many of us are either already there or soon to enter its realm. The strengths and promises of aging are upon us.

The Paradoxes and Paradigms of Old Age

If given the choice to live as long as Madame Calment or Hendrikje van Andel-Schipper, would you take it? When I pose this question to audiences around the country, I often get the same responses: a smattering of enthusiastic takers shoot their hands up right away, but most listeners are more reticent as they sit in contemplation of being so old, wavering their hands back and forth to say "maybe" but with a few hard conditions. "If I kept all my teeth I'd do it," shouted out a middle-aged man at one such event, but then quickly backtracked and added that he would also want to retain the ability to recognize his wife and drive his car if he would ever crest beyond the age of one hundred. Others add similar conditions, such as an intact memory, strong legs, and regular bowel movements among their choices. Within these conditions, I perceive a resignation to the expected decrepitudes of old age and rarely a callout to anything good. My questioning reveals several clear paradoxes of old age: we all want to get there, but we live in fear of what it will entail. We want the best possible old age, but also want to feel and look younger. We rely on the past as the anchor of our identity, yet we must at times let go and break free from it so as to accept and accommodate change. Aging is an inevitable one-way journey and we fret along the way and plot all sorts of manners to stave off or cushion the bumps and blows.

And yet despite some tectonic and wholly positive developments in the life of the average aging person, we are still stuck between two tired and prevalent perspectives on old age: either we must submit gracefully to its rigors and ultimate tragedies, or fight it relentlessly with supposed antiaging strategies until we find a cure. Either way, we are mired in a paradigm that casts old age as our implacable enemy. Even in our designations of successful aging, we view any victories won in daily life as being wrestled away from our inevitably older self. My message here is quite different, however: *aging is the solution and not the problem.* As we all get older, we face inevitable points that pose struggles, losses, reconsiderations, or crises that throw us off balance and force life-altering responses. These age points are as predictable and critically important to our adult development as the milestones of childhood and adolescence. Instead of seeing them as harbingers of decline and old age, however, the seniors that surround me show timeless benefits to aging that emerge and sustain them during these age points, enabling them not simply to cope successfully but also to create new ways of living.

In my previous book on this subject, entitled *How We Age: A Doctor's Journey into the Heart of Growing Old*, I wrote about how we need to place greater value on our elders and hope for a better old age, even in the throes of illness and dementia. My goal was to inspire readers to look at aging in a different and more hopeful vein. But I am not content to simply gaze at the holiness of old age. And neither are the legions of baby boomers and others who are aging by the day. They want to do something and they want to do it now. No more waiting to get old and ill and then die helplessly. No more endless searching for some miraculous antiaging pill that does not exist now and will not exist in the foreseeable future. No more putting hope in antiaging claims that are predictable, tiresome, and largely untrue. The point of this book is to survey the emerging strengths of aging individuals and distill them into a practical, meaningful action plan for a better aging process.

CR

I realize that this mission may prompt some doubts. Whether we consider our own aging self or look to those much older, we see daunting decline and loss. In my geriatric psychiatry practice tending to some of the most ill and debilitated elders, I see the worst forces of old age every day. Despite our deepest yearnings and the billions of dollars spent on health care and antiaging products, no one has escaped aging and everyone will eventually die. As a result, many will argue that any such benefits we imagine in late life are mostly illusory and short-lived at best. There is even a moral argument that we should resist prolonging our life beyond its natural boundaries, so as to clear the brush, so to speak, for successive generations. If we have any independence at the end, let it wield a swift and painless blow and avoid the aching, mindless languishing that so many endure.

Such realism has many prominent voices who will extol aging only up until a certain point. "It's great to be old," says author Susan Jacoby, "as long as one does not manifest too many of the typical problems of advanced age." Longer years may only bring more illness, poverty, and privation to the majority of elders in our youth-focused culture. She calls into question many of the supposed benefits of aging, including the sacrosanct notion of wisdom, and points out the risk in believing that any or all of our supposedly healthy habits will bring a better future. We hit a wall sooner or later when, as Jacoby asserts, "anyone who has outlived his or her passions has lived too long."

Similarly, medical ethicist Ezekiel Emanuel argues that although death is a loss, "living too long is also a loss." In his provocative article "Why I Hope to Die at 75," Emanuel declares that he will engage in no lifesaving or regenerative therapies beyond the age of seventy-five, as he will have achieved his life goals and made his important contributions by then. He does not intend to shorten or end his life after that point, but he sees no tragedy in its demise, declaring that aging limits both our ambitions and expectations, leaving our "memories framed not by our vivacity but by our frailty." Emanuel projects that his post-seventy-five self will be increasingly "feeble, ineffectual, even pathetic."

Many common folk perspectives on aging adhere to this simple and stark paradigm, defined centrally by a future of decline and struggle. Indeed, most aging individuals face severe attenuation of their most cherished abilities. And many of us will not be fortunate enough to avoid the most common and compelling scourge of old age—*dementia*. One undeniable fact, then, must frame and perhaps even counter any discussion of the strengths and benefits of aging: over 50 percent of the population around the age of eighty-five suffers from Alzheimer's disease or other forms of dementia (called *neurocognitive disorders*, in updated parlance), representing a growing epidemic of monstrous social and economic proportions. These cognitive disorders are game changers in late life, robbing us of independence, identity, and the ability to make the meaningful contributions that once defined us throughout our life span. Writer Kent Russell states quite bluntly in his article "We Are Entering the Age of Alzheimer's" that this disease steals our very humanity, creating "mindless, selfless, unreasonable creatures, somehow still looking like human beings. . . . They might as well be headless bodies, up and shambling around." He portrays old age as a zombie apocalypse—a veritable World War G, for geriatric.

These are strong arguments, but they are neither new nor novel. Jacoby and Emanuel are merely restating the words of Roman statesman and philosopher Cicero, who wrote in 44 BCE: "Old age is the final act of life, as of a drama, and we ought to leave when the play grows wearisome, especially if we have had our fill." Remarkably, Russell is describing a diminished old age no different from that portrayed over four thousand years ago in writings by Ptah-Hotep, first minister to Pharaoh Isesi: "The end of life is at hand; old age descendeth [upon me]; feebleness cometh, and childishness is renewed. He [who is old] lieth down in misery every day. The eyes are small; the ears are deaf . . . and he remembereth not yesterday. . . . *These things doeth old age for mankind, being evil in all things* [emphasis added]." We know these things about the aging process, even as they characterize only the downside. At the same time, neither Jacoby nor Emanuel (nor Cicero, for that matter) would argue against the potential benefits of old age. They simply reject the platitudes about aging that lack empirical evidence or that deny or ignore the difficult and enduring struggles that most people face. This is the gauntlet laid down for any and every commentator on old age—myself included.

So, where does this leave us? What are we to do with our biological fate? British researcher and gerontologist Aubrey de Grey and other life extension proponents recoil from these struggles of aging, loudly proclaiming old age to be a horrible disease that must be cured. The main limitation to progress is not only the rudimentary science on aging, de Grey believes, but a fatalistic and defensive "pro-aging trance" that leads people to see aging as a natural and immutable part of being. In contrast, de Grey and a cadre of antiaging advocates argue that we can eventually solve the tragic mystery of old age by learning to re-engineer cellular aging in order to extend the life span indefinitely. Futurist Ray Kurzweil and his colleague Terry Grossman agree, and outline three successive bridges to this future; the first being present-day dietary and health strategies; the second, the impending biotechnology revolution, to rebuild our body; and the third, an anticipated nanotechnology–artificial intelligence revolution, to rebuild our brain. Many young aging people crowd onto this first bridge, enlisting various body and brain exercises and other remedies touted for extending the life span. There are significant merit and considerable science behind some of these existing approaches, but as I emphasized before, they cannot guarantee any individual positive outcome, and practical applications for more radical technological innovations are barely on the radar. This is the enduring uncertainty of aging with which we all live.

In the face of this seemingly inescapable predicament, we continue to frame old age in a narrow and simplistic manner. Such a prevailing model is based on a mechanistic series of steps that inexorably unravel our youth. Biologist and aging researcher Robert Arking casts this journey in corresponding scientific terms, defining aging as a "time-dependent series of cumulative, progressive, intrinsic, and deleterious functional and structural changes that usually begin to manifest themselves at reproductive maturity and eventually culminate in death." This definition is accurate and it is echoed in much of our experience. Beginning around middle age, we take notice of accumulating physical changes, medical issues, and losses. Development gives way to decline, and gains slip away to losses. Dreams of youth seem less attainable. We begin to have more and more experiences in which our aspirations butt up against fading abilities and opportunities.

It is at this very juncture, however, when something *remarkable* may happen that can change the way we view and experience aging, affecting the very meaning of what it is to be old. Aging begins to unfold in a beautiful and yet maddening fashion wholly different from our typical cast of it, bringing not simply glory and destruction, joy and despair, but an incredibly complex weave of these experiences. The result is a powerfully enriching and contagious culture of aging representing an expression of our achieved humanity and an incubator for further growth.

I propose here a different paradigm of aging along with an action plan that identifies and engages the myriad pieces of our own aging self that can dispel negative stereotypes of being "old" and bring renewed hope in our future. This paradigm shows how one can actively live a creative age as opposed to falling headlong into an uncontrollable old. Age must neither define us nor serve as only a limiting, negative factor, but should become a powerful, life-changing tool that enables us to elevate, celebrate, and transcend being old in ways that have profound influences on our personal world and the greater world around us. We can begin to consider the keys to these lifelong explorations and achievements with an interesting thought experiment.

∾

Imagine that you are young again. Some magical potion will transport you down a nostalgic rabbit hole to an age that seems to represent the peak of youth, vigor, and vitality. You can revisit and rewrite your life, making different choices, correcting mistakes, and seeking out the relationships or pursuits you still treasure and those you regret having ignored or left behind. You can make great changes to devise a new future, or attempt to follow the same course that has brought you everything that you value today. It's an impossible but intriguing fantasy that we all engage in from time to time, perhaps increasingly as the years pass by and more of our life lies behind us than ahead.

And yet it is easy to miss an essential element in these musings. Pull back the curtain to reveal the true master behind these ruminations and you will find, unmistakably, your own well-aged self who is pushing the buttons and pulling the levers. It is all the knowledge, experience, maturity, perspective, balance, and wisdom bequeathed by age that enables you to look back with such keen vision on your life. Would you really trade your current persona for your twenty-one-year-old self to make decisions today? You would have youth, but too much else would be missing. We all think we know the formula to better aging because it is pounded into our eyes and ears and inboxes every day: exercise the body and brain; eat right; drink enough water and get enough sleep; don't overdo the sauce or the spice. We believe that this formula will make our body and brain more like those of young people, but none of the extraordinary elders described in this book based his or her lifestyle on these factors. Exercise and other healthy actions may improve our body and enable a longer life, but they bring no guarantee of a better life. *The true formula is age itself.*

Let's turn, then, to the most fundamental questions that must be asked of our aging self. First, why age? What is the gain in it? Second, why survive? What is the point to living in the face of such daunting struggles? Third, why thrive? Isn't it easier to circle the wagons and maintain stability rather than facing the risks of change? The answers can be found in three emerging strengths of age that mitigate losses and guide us forward: wisdom, purpose, and creativity. These strengths underlie a more balanced and inclusive paradigm of aging that enables us to grab hold and shape our own perspectives and experiences. They can be distilled into a practical action plan that is personalized, purpose-driven, and meaningful. They even apply to aged individuals with severe physical and cognitive losses or diseases, who are typically left out of most models of aging. As we explore these strengths, you will see clearly how aging will trump old, emerging as a life force with struggles and triumphs, losses and gifts, but well lived for us and our loved ones, now and in the future.

PART I

Why Age?

An aged man is but a paltry thing,
A tattered coat upon a stick . . .

— W. B. YEATS, "Sailing to Byzantium"

Old age allows us to "wear the days of our life" as a single
garment—a totality, integrated and complete. In this perspec-
tive, aging is precisely the opposite of deconstruction of the self.

—MATIS WEINBERG, *FrameWorks*

Chapter 1

Aging on Trial

It was the fall of my first year as the mental health director at a large long-term care facility. A phone call came in around ten p.m. to the security office, where the director of nursing, Dorothy, just happened to be working late. A calm and somewhat matter-of-fact voice on the line simply said, "Please come up to room 508. My sister just died." It was an unexpected death, and so Dorothy quickly grabbed her stethoscope and the emergency kit, and headed to the room in the assisted living building with a brisk stride, accompanied by Marie, a nursing assistant. When they entered the room, they immediately found the aged woman seated upright in a chair in a serene repose. Approaching closer, they noted a dusky blue color to her face. She did not appear to be breathing. The woman's sister stood nearby with a sad expression on her face and her hands clasped behind her back. A copy of the book *Final Exit* by Derek Humphrey—a well-known guide to suicide—was lying on the adjacent coffee table.

Dorothy and Marie were initially jarred by the scene but quickly got to work. Marie checked for a pulse while Dorothy placed the bell of her stethoscope on the woman's chest and began listening for signs of life. "It's no use," said the sister, hovering nearby. "She passed away peacefully an hour ago, by her own choice." It was clear to Dorothy that any lifesaving procedures were unnecessary. Just as she reached this conclusion, the security supervisor entered the room, surveyed the scene, and immediately called the police. Within minutes, sirens could be heard approaching the location, and soon the room was full of fire rescue personnel and blue-shirted police officers. Amid this scene, the husband sat silently and with a somber demeanor in the connecting bedroom. Dorothy went to comfort him and ask what had happened, but he declined to elaborate, only telling her that he had said his "good-byes."

As news of the suicide filtered through the community the next day, there was general shock and confusion. "Why had she ended her life?" the residents asked. "Was she ill?" they wondered. As the facility's sole psychiatrist, I was particularly concerned about the impact of the suicide on the woman's family as well as on the staff and residents in the building. I learned that the woman was in her late eighties and had recently moved into the assisted living facility with her husband. She had not been seen by me in our medical clinic, let alone by anyone on my staff. No known warning signs, expressions of discomfort or despair, or unusual behaviors had been reported. The whole event seemed to come out of the blue, until the sister and husband revealed the actual story. The woman had become increasingly concerned about memory lapses over the past few years. She was otherwise in good health and had no previous history of depression, anxiety, or any other mental disorder. Eventually she had seen a neurologist who made a provisional diagnosis of Alzheimer's disease. Because the woman believed that a life of certain decline and loss of independence ran counter to everything that she valued, she decided to end her life painlessly and at a time of her own choosing.

The woman planned her death in the same manner she had lived her life: deliberately, decisively, and detail-orientedly. She intended that her denouement should make a personal statement about life, liberty, and what she thought was the right thing to do in the face of inescapable aging. In the months prior to the suicide, she moved into the assisted living facility so that her husband would have a secure place to live after her death. She researched various methods of suicide and settled on the preferred method from *Final Exit*. She did not inform any staff of her plans, but prepared a letter to family and friends, and asked her sister to be present after she passed away.

The police opened a routine investigation due to the nature of the woman's death, but they did not find any cause or circumstance that warranted further concern. The reaction within the community at the entire facility was quite strong, however, and reflected a bevy of emotions. Many staff members and residents were upset and confused by the death, as it had tapped into deep-seated anxieties. Some individuals felt a sense of loss and grief, and wondered how best to help the family. Others felt hurt and angry. They all wanted to understand the reasons for what happened. Given the sensitive nature of the incident and the widespread concern about its impact on the community that worked and lived in the facility, a meeting of the ethics committee was convened to discuss the death and to suggest ways to best move forward.

The proceedings of the ethics committee began with a relatively narrow focus on the causes of suicide in later life and how it has been viewed, debated, and addressed within the larger medical and mental health communities. These were hot-button issues, and so the committee felt that it made sense to open the meeting with a rather dispassionate review of the scientific literature. As I watched the meeting unfold, I took note of the full attendance as all the committee members came from every part of the facility. The incident had clearly struck a nerve among them, and everyone was eager to offer their own thoughts based on both professional training and personal experiences. A social worker opened by describing the woman who took her own life as a well-regarded community activist who had taken many principled stands over time. Indeed, she argued, the woman's identity had rested on her fierce sense of justice, and it was likely that no one—not her husband, family, or doctors—could stop her once she had made up her mind. She was confident, then, that the woman's suicide would have been nearly impossible to prevent. The discussion over the context of this single suicide was calm at first, but then swelled with emotion as it morphed into a debate over more profound and elusive questions that were now on trial: What is the point of aging in the face of certain mental dissolution and death? Is it justified to end one's life under such circumstances? In succession, each attending group weighed in; doctors, nurses, social workers, administrators, and then clergy. Within short order, the friendly spirit of point and counterpoint degenerated into hardened stances and even a few instances of raised voices.

Not surprisingly, the fierce emotions of the meeting precluded a consensus on the deeper issues about aging that were raised and debated. In the weeks that followed, these vexing questions of life and death, aging and endings bounced around the community and then slowly ebbed, taking with them much of their fervent emotional energy. Although it has been over twenty years since then, the whole experience has remained imprinted on my work. Every day I see individuals who face the same daunting diagnosis as had the woman who killed herself, and their conditions and concerns prompt the same essential question of why we should age.

To begin my search for answers, I want to first return to the woman in question and dig a little deeper into her sentiments. I am now much older than when I first weighed the pros and cons of the woman's decision to end her life. So, how do I feel now, much closer to "old age" than before? Since that first year of my practice, I have had the benefit of hearing many more voices, both wise and wounded, all facing the same dilemma. For a moment, I will try to argue the case of the woman who ended her life, in part by giving voice to what I imagine to have been her concerns:

Imagine yourself in my place. I have lived a life of devotion to my family and my causes. I remember the strength of my arms as they lifted and cared for my infants turned toddlers turned school-children. I was wise and thoughtful with them as they matured into teenagers and then adults, always ready to listen intently and without judgment. During the civil rights era, I did not sit on the couch impassively watching grainy TV images of people suffering; I sat at lunch counters with those afflicted and degraded people and absorbed the same indignities and savage racism. These determined and taut muscles that raised my children also lifted up my oppressed neighbors as they fell under the blows of others. I made this world a better place. But it wasn't the force of my body that made the differ-ence, but the spirit and intellect that guided it—that is my true pride. I decide, therefore I am.

Imagine yourself now in my place. My most cherished abilities— my memory recall, word recognition, abstract thinking—are all slowly beginning to fade. Each day, there is another blow. My body and brain are betraying me and I am furious! Now I have learned that this slide is not temporary and there is no fix; it will grow worse with time to the point where I will lose all sense of my identity and will be completely reliant on the care of others. I will likely cry out unintelligibly, fight the children I raised but no longer recognize, slop all over and soil myself without control, without dignity, and with-out my own voice. My true self will be stilled, replaced by a mindless oppressor who will force my husband, family, and community to care for me, pay for me, and put up with me.

So, why age? Why accept this fate? I choose not to. I know that my life will end, as all lives will eventually end. But I will decide when. I will decide my fate as I always have. That is my strength and my essence.

These words, as I imagine them, are prompted in part by terror of the long and tragic decline faced by our older protagonist. Everything that she held dear seemed to be at risk of total collapse. It was an agonizing situation that demanded a search for some way out. It is hard not to have some understanding for her sentiments, even if our own actions under similar circumstances might not be so bold or calculating.

As we age, all of us face multiple points like this woman reached, where our normal expectations and abilities seem to fail us in the face of a major stress or challenge and we struggle to act and maintain hope. The core stressor may be an injury or illness, a major loss of a loved one or life role, or a natural disaster that saps our strengths and resources. At these points we may feel, at first, that we lack the ability to cope, adjust, and respond. I call these decisive circumstances *age points* and assert that they are the key milestones in our adult life that help determine the forms and the outcomes— the sowing and the reaping—of our own aging self.

From the perspective of the woman who killed herself, her autonomy and integrity were her most precious assets and provided purpose for her daily existence. In the face of losing them, her life had no meaning and she made her exit. She anticipated an old age as portrayed by ethicist Ezekiel Emanuel, in which we slowly but steadily become defined by weakness and decrepitude—a *pathetic* state in which others are inclined to feel sadness or pity in our presence. This attitude assumes an aged life of perpetual and tragic loss even under the best of circumstances, and clearly refuses to balance out the bad with anything good or redeeming. It focuses on the pain and suffering of illness and loss and lets those states trump any relief or remedy that might mitigate the situation. Emanuel has stated that he will not actually kill himself as he ages beyond a certain point, but he will not actively position any fingers in the dike to slow the stream of old age. Of course, this assertion is easier said than done when not actually facing pain and suffering. My own observation after nearly a quarter-century of doctoring is that most people will not only try to plug the hole but search desperately for newer, better solutions. Nonetheless, we must acknowledge the struggles of getting old and decide for ourself our own "whys" of aging.

Why Age?

Why is this question of "why age?" so important? We all age whether we like it or not, so why do we need to justify it, put it on trial and argue for its merits? Just do it and let things fall as they may, one might argue. It's a fair point and perhaps one day all arguments will be rendered moot by an actual Fountain of Youth formula (although then we will contend with much longer lives, which will raise their own enormously complicated personal and societal issues!). This question is so important because we all will face it in various and evolving forms as it pops up through midlife and beyond, sometimes in spoonfuls or cupfuls and other times in bucketfuls when we face crises of ability, strength, morality, or loss. Ultimately, it's a question that taps into the meaning and mission of our life.

A common but misleading assumption underlying this question is that aging is something inherently bad or evil because it diminishes us and leads to our death, a perspective bracketed by the ancient admonition of Ptah-Hotep that old age is "evil in all things" and the modern assertion by Aubrey de Gray that aging is "really bad for you." We may dress it up in many ways, but the bottom line is that the journey has an end that we do not understand. Is it yet possible, then, to develop a counterargument to this—a justification for aging that finds purpose in its process? This search reminds me of the enduring philosophical and theological question about why a divinely created world would allow for evil—the precursor to the modern-day question of why bad things happen to good people. Nineteenth-century German philosopher Gottfried Leibniz was particularly concerned about this issue and developed his *theodicy*, or justification of evil, by positing that we live in the best of all possible worlds that God could create, and that even evil has a higher, albeit hidden function in this divine perfection. By extension, perhaps we need our own *gerodicy*, or justification, for aging that sees it as either a naturally or divinely ordained process that unfolds in its own meaningful and necessary ways. Fortunately, there are several essential and compelling reasons for why we ought to age.

Aging Helps Us Survive

Although we take as a given our existence as creatures that get old and die, there are other pathways in the cosmos of living things. The tiny box-shaped jellyfish *Turritopsis dohrnii*, for example, lives a potentially immortal life oscillating between spore and adult, and then back again. The quaking aspen trees in Colorado's Trembling Giant grove will sprout, grow tall, and then die over an average 130-year cycle, but their massive living root base has been around for over eighty thousand years. The evolutionary path of humans, however, has been quite different. Our primeval ancestors were likely small shrewlike creatures that lived a short and precarious

life among the dinosaurs, with natural selection driving their continued existence only through rapid reproductive success. Old age
didn't exist in an environment that had no use for individuals beyond the stage of reproduction and basic rearing. Any slowing or
weakening in the body of these progenitors hastened their journey to the jaws of a multitoothed meat-eater. In this world, nature
didn't need old age for anything other than a reliable food supply!
In and of itself, aging had no purpose.

These small mammals emerged from their dens following the
great extinction of the dinosaurs and flourished, evolving over
millions of years into a multitude of mammals, including *Homo
sapiens*. Still, old age would seem to have no purpose in a world
that was only marginally safer than that of previous epochs. Natural selection favored genes that passed themselves along by improving and increasing reproduction. The evolutionary theory of
aging suggests that natural selection would not favor the accumulation of any genes for longevity nor would it weed out mutations
that hasten aging, since they would have no bearing on reproductive success. Some genes might accumulate that cause negative effects later in life as long as they benefit development earlier in life.
In the rough-and-tumble world of early humans, one might even
argue that old people would burden the tribe by competing for
resources needed by young people to thrive and multiply. From
this vantage point, the clan with young, nimble, and short-lived
members might reproduce and thrive more than would the tribe
weighted down by age. In this world, old age would seem to have
no advantage.

With the emergence of modern humankind, however, the
calculus of aging changed. Age brought greater accumulation of
knowledge and experience, so that the elders of the clan, tribe, or
village were the key repositories of essential know-how. Anthropologist Tanya Luhrmann described these old folks to me as critical

contributors to survival. Psychiatrist George Vaillant has called them "Keepers of the Meaning" and "Guardians." They were the medicine men and women, the shamans and the tribal leaders; they knew where to find the necessary medicinal plants, how to conjure the spirits, when to foment battle and when to seek peace. There were the ancient search engines, the gray-haired apps who set the direction and cohesion of the community. Even evolutionary biologists have reconsidered the value of these older members, suggesting that they may actually increase overall reproductive success in a group by helping younger parents rear a higher number of healthier offspring. This phenomenon, dubbed the "grandmother hypothesis," has been seen in studies of orcas and pilot whales as well as in anthropological studies of humans. So, in answering our question of "why age?" science both savages and saves us: we are weaker and less reproductive as we get older, but the accumulated fruits of our presence and our direct intergenerational contributions provide a key reserve of energy and wisdom.

Aging Brings Wisdom

If our aging body can provide some value for survival, how about our aging spirit? I decided to pursue this question of "why age" by surveying several religious leaders who are themselves aging and tending to enormous flocks of aging congregants. My first stop was Rabbi Solomon Schiff, who was, in my estimation, the unofficial rabbi of Miami since he led the Rabbinical Association of Greater Miami for over forty years. He has been involved with my own institution for the entirety of his fifty-eight years in Miami—serving as one of the official clergy members as well as being a sought-after advisor. I have known Rabbi Schiff for over eighteen years but our family lineages were intertwined nearly a century ago. His father studied at the famous yeshiva in Lomza, Poland, in the early

1900s, certainly under the tutelage of my maternal great-great-grandfather, who was a beloved teacher of the Torah and other sacred Jewish texts at the same school. So, now the teaching came full circle, and I sat with Rabbi Schiff one afternoon in my office to ask what he has learned about why we age from both Judaism and his own eighty-seven years.

Rabbi Schiff has a special gift to conjure up a story or a joke relevant to any topic presented to him—what in Yiddish he calls *zalts un fefer* (salt and pepper)—and he uses this skill to spice up any sermon or discourse with interesting tidbits and stories. He began our discussion on why we age, then, with a little seasoning regarding the patriarch Abraham. "It is written in the Torah that 'Abraham became old' after his wife Sarah died. So, what does this mean?" the rabbi began. "We know he lived a long life, but why did he suddenly age?" According to legends from the Talmud, the rabbi continued, there were once no outward signs of old age, and so a father and a son—Abraham and Isaac, for example—could be mistaken for each other. So, Abraham petitioned God that old age would have a certain appearance to distinguish it. "And why," the rabbi inquired, "would we want to look older, especially today when we spend billions of dollars trying to look younger? I will tell you why: if you cannot see the difference between one generation and the next, how will the younger ones know who has more experience, knowledge, and wisdom?" God made us age so that we can be symbols of wisdom.

I followed up my theological question with a personal one, asking the rabbi what he himself has learned from his own eighty-seven years about the whys of aging and the meaning of the wisdom God grants us. "I have become more tolerant and accepting of other people and their different points of view. I feel a greater sense of obligation in my remaining years to teach others and to help them look for the good in other people. It says in *Pirke Avot* [The Sayings of Our Fathers] that one should judge all people on the good side, and give them the benefit of the doubt. I feel closer to this as I move along the road of life."

Whether one reads the Bible as a Jew or Christian, the text is replete with aged characters who lived extraordinarily long and active lives. I was curious, then, whether a rabbi and a Catholic priest would have any differences in opinion. Rabbi Schiff suggested I speak to his friend Miami archbishop Thomas Wenski. I was glad for the introduction, and within weeks of my question I met with the rabbi and archbishop in his office at the Miami Archdiocese headquarters on Biscayne Boulevard. These two men of God have known each other for many years, and both are funny, gregarious, and thoughtful men, happy to talk about aging—and although they emphasize different holy books, they are mostly on the same page.

The sixty-seven-year-old archbishop, like the rabbi, referenced his own aged wisdom: "I've gotten more patient—I've mellowed," he told me, extraordinary for a man in charge of one of the largest and most diverse archdioceses in the country and whose plate is replete with vexing challenges and controversies. One of these directly touches aging, as priests face mandatory retirement at age seventy-five and Wenski must sometimes sound the bell for one reluctant to step aside. "It's a difficult transition for them," he said: "fear of the unknown, loss of role, and a reckoning with what to do with oneself." And yet Wenski and his priests have a supreme role model of aging in Pope Benedict XVI, who retired in 2013 due to failing health and the overwhelming demands of the papacy. Father Benedict, as he prefers to be called now, still writes and attends Vatican events. He was able to serenely relinquish control of one of the world's most influential positions and pursue his remaining years in relative piety and solitude. It is an impressive and inspiring model of aging.

In terms of my direct question on the "whys" of aging, the arch-bishop referenced the thinking of his own master, Pope Francis, as written in a wonderful interreligious dialogue on faith. Pope Francis equates aging with the practical benefit of wisdom, and cites a passage from the Book of Kings in which King Solomon's son Rehoboam assumes the throne and first seeks advice from the older men who served his father and who counsel kindness and forbearance to his people. Unfortunately, the new king "forsook the counsel of the old men . . . and took counsel with the young men that were grown up with him," and they instructed him to be harsh and uncompromising with the people. The result was a revolt of many tribes and the breakup of the kingdom of Israel. Both rabbi and priest nodded in agreement to the core message of this story; aging brings wisdom that is essential to the unity and progress of both the spirit and the community, and one forsakes it at his or her own peril.

Like its sibling faiths, Islam also places great value on both aging and the aged. Imam Naseeb Khan, leader of a mosque serving the same South Florida communities as those of Rabbi Schiff and Archbishop Wenski, noted that Islamic traditions accord an increasing degree of respect and family obligations with each year of life, along with the commandment to be kind and gracious to someone older. Aging is particularly "lauded and respected," said Khan, because it is seen not as a "deficiency but as wisdom." This focus on respect for aging and the role of the aged as wise is also prescribed in Hinduism, where the ancient text of the Bhagavad Gita describes a multitude of wise attributes that we gain with time. Confucian thought stipulates filial piety as a fundamental obligation to honor, respect as well as care for the elderly. Similarly, in Buddhism there is great respect for the aging person.

My source for a Buddhist answer to "why age?" was Buddhist priest and author Lewis Richmond. Born of a Jewish father and a

Greek Orthodox mother, Richmond was raised as a Unitarian but became a Buddhist after encountering a Buddhist teacher while studying in a Unitarian seminary. In our discussion, we discovered that we share a common root in our intellectual lineages, as we both took a college course with Erik Erikson on his life cycle theory—Lewis in 1967 when Erikson was at the peak of his career, and I in 1984 when he was in its twilight, suffering from dementia. Regardless of his state of mind, Erikson was equally inspiring and influential on our thinking.

Lewis pointed out that when Buddhism was first developed over two thousand years ago, the average life expectancy was short and life was rough. This environment nurtured dual perspectives in Buddhist thinking: life is certainly fleeting, but this makes it all the more precious and beautiful. The purpose of aging is no different than the purpose of living, and so aging carries no distinction of being less worthy. Quite the contrary: aging is not about getting weaker, but is a journey of finding greater value and enlightenment or wisdom. Buddhist philosophy teaches us to respect, appreciate, and care equally for young and old lives.

Lewis's own philosophy at the age of sixty-nine was profoundly shaped by his surviving both cancer and a near fatal bout of encephalitis in his midfifties. These health crises reinforced his belief in the preciousness of life, and the desire to freely pursue his dreams. Buddhism taught him that there is a fluidity to one's identity, and that "every breath" brings "new chances." These beliefs gave him the confidence and freedom to start over and reinvent his life. Now that he is semiretired from his role as a Buddhist priest and software entrepreneur, Lewis has started several new pursuits as a piano teacher, a mentor for other writers, and a musician and composer with his new band. Lewis has learned that despite our physical decline with age, there is not the same straight-line decline in our mental capacities. Certain kinds of mental skills even improve with age, such as the ability to solve a problem based on experience and the integration of information, a quality best defined as *wisdom*.

Aging Brings Positivity and Purpose

The way in which we think about and perceive aging can have an important impact on how aging unfolds. All too often, however, we are schooled in a negative paradigm. At a recent fiftieth birthday celebration for one of my friends, the assembled group presented him with "Dr. D. Crepit's Over the Hill Survival Kit" consisting of a mock doctor's bag picturing a balding, loony caricature of an old man in a white coat and containing a package of "50 Sucks" lollipops and the "Old Geezer Lost Yer Marbles Replacement Pack." Everyone got a good laugh at age's expense, but it made me wonder: How would we react to a similar gag gift that denigrated one's gender, ethnicity, or religious identity? No doubt it would be highly offensive and would be pilloried by party-goers. But here it was perfectly accepted and enjoyed, with age somehow being a fair target for such put-downs. And therein lies the problem: we reflexively define aging by its downside. There is great risk that such a pervasive, negative narrative of aging becomes a self-fulfilling prophecy.

In fact, psychologist Becca Levy has shown that we may actually become what we believe about aging, good or bad. Her "stereotype embodiment theory" posits that age stereotypes can become internalized and have an unconscious but profound impact on performance, health, and longevity. If you see yourself as age impaired, your performance on memory, handwriting, and mathematical tests can be shaded in negative ways. In a similar finding, Ellen Langer's "counterclockwise" study of older men showed that immersion in an environment that reminded them of younger days and forced them to think and act like their younger self had a significantly positive impact on their overall health and function in just a few weeks.

More profoundly, Levy found that people with positive self-perceptions about aging—attitudes that have roots in what they learn as young and middle-aged adults—demonstrate median survival rates 7.5 years longer than do those with negative self-perceptions. Data from the Baltimore Longitudinal Study on Aging provide one likely explanation for this finding. Those individuals with more negative ratings on the Attitudes Toward Older People Scale had twice the rate of cardiovascular events, such as heart attacks and strokes. In contrast, individuals with a significantly positive attitude toward aging had an 80 percent reduction in cardiovascular events. Similarly, data from various parts of the Middle Age in the United States (MIDUS) Study has shown that having a sense of purpose is also associated with reducing cardiovascular and other causes of mortality.

How do we get such positive and purposeful attitudes? Aging! The aging brain has been shown to shift its focus onto more positive images, beliefs, and attitudes. Psychologist Laura Carstensen's "socioemotional selectivity theory" attributes these age-related changes to our realization in later life that our life span is shorter and we are better served by engaging in activities or relationships that are more emotionally meaningful and satisfying. Imagine, for example, that you have only a few more days to live. What would you do? Some people might crawl up in a ball and await their ending, but many others would instinctively gather around them the most important people, personal effects, and foods so as to maximize the meaning and pleasure of those last moments. The aging process, whether measured in years or decades, brings a more drawn out but similar situation as we develop a keener vision of the horizon of our life span. Aging itself becomes the motivation to improve both the quality and quantity of life.

What Happens When We Get Too Old?

The greatest challenge to finding our "whys" of aging is the accumulating and inevitably overwhelming impact of physical decline, disease, losses of loved ones, and impending death, which cut into the marrow of our existence. We all become physically and aesthetically diminished with age. We are orphaned when we lose our parents and the other individuals who loved us the most. We are bereft of these cherished creators of our original worlds—and hence of the worlds themselves. We are threatened with the possibility of feeling unloved and unwanted. We imagine and anticipate our own death and wonder what the point will have been to our life if nothingness arrives. As age-associated changes accumulate, there may come an eventual tipping point in which our daily life becomes determined by chronic and progressive conditions, such as bone loss and joint degeneration, severe visual and hearing loss, and dementia, which can cause immobility, pain, isolation, disillusionment, and confusion. Even with the best of health care, these conditions will limit the essential activities and joys of our aging self.

The psychoanalyst Erik Erikson and his wife, Joan, tried to capture this final stage of life by adding a new, ninth stage to Erik's life cycle theory. Erikson had previously laid out a captivating notion of eight stages of life from birth to old age, with each unfolding stage characterized by a tension between having to exercise and develop specific strengths at the risk of flailing or even failing due to absent or underdeveloped skills. These acquired strengths (or weaknesses) build upon one another and propel our development.

Erikson initially limited old age to the eighth stage, in which there is a tension between establishing a sense of integrity for one's accomplishments and assets versus feeling despairing over one's failed efforts or diminishing opportunities. Beyond this stage, however, lies a time typically in one's eighties and nineties (or in younger years due to catastrophic medical or psychiatric conditions) where debility and uncertainty may have the upper hand. As their theory (and life circumstances) evolved, the Eriksons described this period as a *ninth* stage where "hope may easily give way to despair in the face of continued and increasing disintegration, and in light of both chronic and sudden indignities. Even the simple activities of daily living may present difficulty and conflict."

This ninth stage is the potential monster in the closet, the "evil" and the "bad" of old age in which we might heartily agree with Emanuel and others who rail against any attempts to sew a silk purse from the rotted sow's ear. I will describe the ninth stage vividly in a single afternoon of seeing my patients. First there is Barbara, an eighty-five-year-old widow who lives with unremitting pain from severe degenerative joint disease. She is depressed, nervous, and hopeless. Then there is Edgar, a seventy-eight-year-old man who has no short-term memory and is unable to speak due to advanced Alzheimer's disease. He is confused, frightened, and angry. Maricela is ninety, nearly blind, physically frail, and poor. She lives alone and is severely depressed. These individuals face enormous daily struggles and heartaches, and seem to prompt a justification for never wanting to be found in such circumstances and for seeking a handy way out if they should occur. The earlier-described woman who killed herself pulled the rip cord before hitting the terminal velocity of the ninth stage. Would you do the same?

Contemplate such a future for a moment, but then return to our basic questions: Why age? Where is the gain in it? Could aging bring strengths even in the ninth stage? Sometimes the right formula can stabilize and bolster these individuals. I have seen the stunning rejuvenation of aged individuals when newfound love or purpose comes along. Even a tiny glimmer of hope combined with the recruitment of social supports can buffer and sometimes transform the profound loss and grief of such individuals as Barbara, Edgar, and Maricela. For example, Barbara finally agreed to enroll in a pain rehab program, and after intensive physical therapy and medication adjustment, she was walking (and smiling) with less pain and feeling rejuvenated. Edgar was enrolled in a music program and started on medication for depression; within weeks he was a calmer and more contented man. Maricela was enrolled in a community program that provided health care and a day program of activities at a center near her home. Her health and overall well-being improved significantly as she connected with others and got basic help with meals and medications. No rocket science was needed here, but each person required help from committed individuals who took the time to see what he or she needed and then marshalled the appropriate resources and connections. Once the roadblocks were removed, the age-given strengths of each person began to emerge and shine.

Another Death, but Different

During the summer of my eighteenth year as the director of mental health at a large long-term care facility, an older woman died one evening. Unlike the sudden and tumultuous suicide of the woman discussed earlier, this death was not unexpected. Janet had suffered from Alzheimer's disease for the past seven years. In the days leading up to her passing, her loving husband, children, and grandchildren all came to assemble around her bed, hold her hands, caress her, and speak to her lingering presence. I had stepped into the room a few hours before she died, to hover by her slumbering form and reflect on the journey. I tried to imagine her sentiments and put them into words, starting at the same point as with our earlier, exit-seeking woman:

Imagine yourself in my place. *I come from a family of determined and creative immigrants who were the first generation in my family to leave China and make a life in America. I remember sharing a room with my grandmother when I was ten years old. She was an old woman to everyone but me, since I could only see her strength and warmth. I learned to bake and to quilt from my mother and other beloved elders. They showed me how to work hard and keep on working, no matter the circumstances. The undaunted spirit that they brought to this country is woven into the fiber of my being.*

Continue to imagine yourself in my place. *Something is wrong with me now. I can't always find the words I try to conjure. There are blank spots in my days. Maybe I am becoming like my mother and her father in their later years, struggling to remember. No matter. There is work to be done and I am needed by my family and others. There is a little girl at our church suffering from cancer and I must complete this quilt in the next two days so she can hold it tightly in her hands when she begins treatment. Let the fruits of my own hands strengthen her. I quilt, therefore I am.*

I still wake up every morning with a recipe in my head waiting to be baked. Today will be my mother's poppy-seed cake. Perhaps tomorrow it's a day for lemon squares. I bake, therefore I am.

I am still a mother to my children and a wife to my husband. My daughter cried today as we packed up my bags to move into a new place. I am not certain why I am going there, but go I must, like when my grandmother set out from China to Detroit. I held my

daughter close as I've always done, and I told her: "It's time. Life
changes. I must accept this."
From out of my fog this mother still rises.

In the years of her life after being diagnosed with Alzheimer's
disease, Janet's path did, at many moments, encompass the very
difficult and agonizing symptoms I envision frightening anyone
suffering from dementia. But there were also many if not more
moments of joy and connection with Janet's family that enlivened
her spirit and brought purpose even in her depths. Her life both
before and after her diagnosis was like the stunning quilt she created and which was pictured on the program from her funeral—
shaped by beautiful vines covered with multicolored leaves and
flowing in endless circles. Like Janet and her entire world from
start to finish, there was harmony and purpose in its stitching.

A Verdict for the Trial on Aging

In my search for answers to the question of why we should age, I've
tried to part the clouds a bit to reveal that aging brings strengths.
This fact will not satisfy everyone, and one might still believe that
there is no good to aging beyond a certain point. My fear is that in
neglecting to preserve and enrich an aging life, whether our own
or that of others, we send a message that life only has meaning
when we are happy, comfortable, and independent. These are essential goals that we reach in fits and starts, but achieving them
seems shaky if we only look to fate. We have the ability and the
responsibility, instead, to make choices to be open and accepting
of life circumstances, to search out answers and to create new ones,
and to connect with and do for others. We can choose to end the

pejorative notion of old that haunts us and instead make aging into something better for ourself and for those in the ninth stage who have more limited abilities and choices.

The two women who bookend this trial took very different pathways at a critical age point: one woman chose not to go on, whereas the other simply moved forward as best she good, diminished but still determined. Our own aging life may or may not be framed by something as consequential as dementia, but there will certainly be other age-related factors, and we will have to find ways to move forward and to search for the good in the process. Science and religion provide one fundamental answer: aging brings a broadening of our knowledge, roles, and vision that can be encompassed by the term wisdom. This wisdom is based upon and fueled by fundamental reserves of brain connections, skills, social instincts, emotional and spiritual maturity, and creative powers that continue to grow and develop with age. Even in the ninth stage, this reserve of wisdom plays important roles, when presence can substitute for performance and the process of connection can substitute for productivity. Janet's life illustrated these strengths, as her knowledge of family recipes, her enduring creative skills, and her roles in the family continued to enrich her own life and that of so many others. Her legacy, which was forged as much in her aging years as in her younger ones, is clearly imprinted across three generations. Even for the woman who ended her life, there was a powerful reserve of wisdom that was cut short. By examining these lives, we discover how even when our daily existence appears painful, muddled, and teetering, the forces of wisdom can bring an unspoken and transcendent sense of possibility, purpose, and hope.

Chapter 2

Building Reserve, Using Wisdom

A life honorably and virtuously led . . . can crown old age with this blessed harvest of its past labors.

—CICERO, "On Old Age"

FOR SEVERAL YEARS, I was the visiting psychiatrist at a residential facility called Palm Haven for older adults with chronic mental illnesses, such as schizophrenia. It was an unassuming, two-story building nestled in a quiet Miami neighborhood and surrounded by towering live oaks and cabbage palm trees that obscured its corners and shaded an inner courtyard where the residents sat to relax, chat, and smoke between activities and at dusk. The three dozen residents were men and women in their late fifties through eighties who came to the program after years of bouncing between psychiatric hospitals, transient apartments, and the street. They constituted an amazingly varied group whose histories read like episodes from *Survivorman*. Eduardo, for example, was a seventy-two-year-old man with chronic paranoid schizophrenia who lived off snails, bugs, and assorted plants along the canals of South Florida for several years before coming to Palm Haven. Susan was an eighty-year-old woman who was rescued from a burning apartment fire set by her own madness, and then committed to a locked state hospital for over a decade. Frankie was a sixty-seven-year-old former jazz musician who played in small clubs throughout the rural South until his schizophrenia made him think that his trumpet was an instrument of the devil. Now in their later years, they all lived together relatively harmoniously under the direction of Dr. Michaels, an energetic and devoted psychologist nicknamed "Queen Mermaid" by Frankie.

The symptoms of schizophrenia are well known to most clinicians: severe and mentally debilitating delusions and hallucinations; disorganized speech and behavior; and an array of disturbances in mood, social function, and volition. Case by case, however, schizophrenia is a coat of many colors in which the symptomatic picture is as varied as the number of individuals with the disease. With improvements in both psychiatric and medical care, more individuals with schizophrenia are experiencing a longer, healthier life span. A certain percentage demonstrates less florid psychosis but more social withdrawal, apathy, and cognitive dulling that comes with age and correlates with increased loss of brain tissue.

I must confess that I held a certain amount of trepidation before my arrival to Palm Haven. The treatment of schizophrenia is challenging, especially with older individuals who are afflicted with an additional layer of age-associated medical problems and physical disabilities. Most of the residents' medication regimens defied any established algorithm, and consisted of tangled webs of oral and injectable antipsychotics, mood stabilizers, antidepressants, and hypnotics, in addition to pills for high blood pressure, heart disease, and various other maladies. It was a daunting task to apprehend each resident's history and treatment course, and so I readied myself for many long afternoons in the small conference room at Palm Haven, where I met with the residents each week.

What I encountered was quite different from what I imagined. To be certain, the residents were still struggling with residual symptoms. At the same time, lifelong manifestations of psychosis had receded in many of them, and they were more engaged in life than ever before. Living in a stable and supportive environment and participating in therapeutic activities had an impact. The key was to look behind each appearance and see the entirety of the underlying person. For example, one of the residents named Dorothy had severe abnormal movements of her tongue and facial muscles from years of taking antipsychotic medications that literally disfigured her and frightened people away. Yet, sitting and talking with her, I encountered an incredibly friendly and gracious woman who was sociable, empathic, and devoted to her family. And then there was wide-eyed Oliver, with his hair tousled into permanent bedhead and every area of exposed skin—mouth, cheeks, and fingers—awash in yellow tobacco stain. Oliver spoke in a loud, growling monotone that sometimes betrayed a residual southern drawl. In his aging years at Palm Haven he evolved from a maniacal-appearing chain smoker to a softer, more engaged man who wrote poetry, composed songs, and was eager to relate his family history through a series of photo albums he previously had kept secreted away in a duffle bag.

My impressions of such patients as Dorothy and Oliver are supported by the work of my fellow geriatric psychiatrist Dr. Dilip Jeste, one of America's foremost experts on late-life schizophrenia. Early in his career he also observed that some aging individuals with schizophrenia got better with time, and not just because they were the healthiest and heartiest of the bunch who survived longer. Instead, he believed that they improved because they developed more insight and took active roles to improve their conditions. In addition, Jeste saw how aging helped these individuals develop such strengths as wisdom, resilience, and optimism. Intrigued by these emerging strengths of age, he decided to study the concept of wisdom at a time when hardly a mention appeared in the psychiatric literature. He began by looking to his own roots in India.

As a young boy living in the city of Pune in western India, Jeste was enthralled with James Hilton's 1933 novel *Lost Horizon*, which tells the story of several British characters who are spirited away to the fictional village of Shangri-La. Hidden high in the Himalayas, Shangri-La shelters its inhabitants in a warm and lush valley where they routinely live to several hundred years of age in health and happiness. Although he was disappointed to learn that *Lost Horizon* was only a story, the vision of a better aging always stuck with Jeste and was echoed throughout his life. He grew up surrounded by vibrant aged role models, such as his uncle and grandfather, who exposed him to Indian plays, concerts, and politics, and later, his psychiatric mentor Dr. N. S. Vahia, who was renowned as one of the fathers of modern psychiatry in India.

Positive views on aging also flowed from his Hindu religion and culture. One of the most popular Hindu deities in Jeste's home state of Maharashtra is the elephant-headed Ganesha, the god of wisdom and knowledge and the remover of obstacles. Each year, millions of dancing devotees carry colorful garland-wrapped statues of Ganesha in processions through the streets of Mumbai to their eventual dunking in nearby waterways. Jeste applied the spirit of Ganesha to aging, advocating that we continue to learn and gain wisdom so as to optimize success and remove age-associated obstacles from our paths. He mined the sacred Hindu scripture of the Bhagavad Gita for its commentaries on wisdom and found a multitude of descriptions, ranging from knowledge to self-control to insight and humility. He learned how many other religions had similar conceptualizations of wisdom. Across every dimension of his life, then—from his upbringing, religion, culture, and scientific studies—Jeste saw how the aging process develops unique strengths.

In many ways, Palm Haven was Miami's hidden Shangri-La for its residents with debilitating and progressive psychiatric conditions who were getting better with age. Their courses reminded me of the well-known story of John Nash, the Nobel Prize–winning mathematician featured in the movie *A Beautiful Mind,* whose brilliant academic career was cut short by the onset of paranoid schizophrenia, but who emerged later in life with fewer symptoms and a renewed ability to study and teach. Such individuals portray a fascinating paradox of aging: our body and brain decline in clearly measurable ways, and yet our functioning as a whole may remain stable or even improve in other ways. If aging can bring improvement even in some individuals struggling with chronic mental illness, we can only imagine the strengths it can bring to those with a more stable mind! How do we explain this paradox and then leverage its positive elements?

How Aging Helps

Aging would seem, at first, to be the enemy of the brain. Studies that measure brain size on MRI scans show slow but steady loss of brain tissue starting in our early thirties and with an acceleration after the age of sixty. This process is revealed in microscopic views of aging brains that show declining numbers of brain cells or neurons and the increasing presence of frayed nerve connections and proteinaceous plaques. These changes vary in their trajectory over time depending on which region of the brain is examined, but become more common with advancing age and can be matched directly to specific mental changes. The picture is even bleaker in neurocognitive disorders, such as Alzheimer's disease, in which there is an explosion of abnormal protein deposits both inside and outside of neurons that slow their metabolism, sever their connections to other cells, choke off their blood supply, and ultimately kill them. Just looking at the average aging brain, then, will not bring much optimism.

Most of us are well aware of the changes in our brain's abilities as we age into our fifties and beyond. On the one hand, our knowledge, skills, and ability to communicate with others remain relatively stable and continue to develop and improve with increasing experience. We call this our *crystallized intelligence* and it is our base, our pride, and the foundation for all that we do in our lives well into our eighties and nineties. At the same time, most of us notice that memory recall seems more sluggish, tip-of-the-tongue memory lapses become more common, and multitasking is more difficult. We are less efficient at sifting through the daily stream of information and suppressing distracting stimuli, leading us to be more selective in how many things we choose to focus on and tackle. These skills underlie our powers of reasoning, problem-solving, and pattern recognition, which make up our *fluid intelligence*, and they all undergo more predictable and dramatic declines as we cross middle age and progress into later life. Put on a curve, both fluid and crystallized skills show variable arcs of change, but each with inevitable downward slopes as we age into our eighties and nineties.

Too often we write the story of aging based on these cognitive changes, assuming that our mind follows the same pathway as our body—slowing, breaking down, and eventually failing as we dissipate into dementia. We cast ourselves as the loony white-haired codger on the gag gift my friend received on his fiftieth birthday—hysterical, disconnected, and in need of more "marbles." It's a portrayal of aging as ugly as any racist or sexist attitude that we would otherwise soundly reject. Despite its widespread acceptance, however, there are several fundamental reasons that explain why this model of brain aging is both distorted and misleading:

We are more complex: Our average performance across several limited and artificial cognitive tests does not capture the variability and complexity of our abilities in real-world situations. For example, there are many resourceful and creative people who just happen to score low on standardized tests of mathematical ability. Test-taking deficits don't wipe out our other positive abilities.

Slow ≠ worse: A "slower" performance does not equal a "worse" performance, since the lesser speed of the aged mind might simply be reflecting a different approach that is equal or even better in form and outcome. For example, young and nimble brains can read sentences that are interrupted with distracting text more rapidly than can older, slower brains, but the older brains tend to have greater comprehension of what is written.

It misses our strengths: Many age-developed strengths, such as wisdom and creativity, are difficult to measure but are certainly present and have profoundly positive impact.

We can compensate: Our mind and brain can buffer losses by drawing upon our vast reserves of brainpower.

Consider instead how aging may bring improvement in thinking and behaving by answering the same question I posed in the introduction: When do you think you made better decisions—when you were twenty-one years old or now? We might first believe that younger ages always have the advantage since they bring peak performance of both brain and body, with our youthful energy ready to conquer the world and be fruitful and multiply. In turn, we imagine that we need to train our older brain to be more like younger brains. However, most of us instinctively know the real answer as to when we make better decisions: *Now*, of course! And why? Logically and practically speaking, aging changes us in fundamental ways that age twenty-one can't touch:

- *Time* brings us an accumulation of *knowledge*, experience, and skills.
- We learn *lessons* from trial and error that enhance our *judgment* and force us to persevere in the face of adversity.
- *Failure* leads to humility, gratitude, *empathy*, and healthy dependence on others.
- *Ambition* and a desire for *legacy* motivates us to build, compose, and *create* new things.
- The *approach of death* reshuffles our priorities and brings us increased *insight* and a transcendent perspective on life.

The experience of aging and only aging, then, helps us perpetually develop five core strengths: knowledge, judgment, empathy, creativity, and insight. Our ability to make the most practical and beneficial decisions depends upon and grows with these elements. Put together, they compose the greatest gift of aging: *wisdom*.

Wisdom as a Five-Pointed Crown

If you want to protect your finances and plan for retirement or a major catastrophe, you are wise to keep a diversified reserve of assets. Similarly, our aging brain develops a protective reserve as a form of physical and mental insurance that enables us to continue functioning in the face of damage, disease, and dysfunction. Such a reserve sets the threshold for what we can bear before noticeable decline sets in. It enables us to compensate, reroute, and even grow new capacities through a process called neuroplasticity. It banks a broad set of intellectual, emotional, and spiritual experiences and abilities that we can activate when needed in the form of a vital and ever expanding mental energy known as wisdom.

Our common notion of wisdom tends to be limited and stereotyped. It's King Solomon sitting on his throne and deciding how to split an infant between two battling mothers. It's a white-bearded man or a long-haired and shawled older lady spouting aphorisms on the good life. Sometimes it's simply portrayed as an owl wearing spectacles and a mortarboard. These symbols imply that wisdom is associated with being old, wide-eyed, and imbued with some great or transcendent power, but they do not really tell us what wisdom is all about. In a general sense, we can define wisdom as the ability to deftly apply our accumulated knowledge and experience to decision making. Paul Baltes's influential Berlin wisdom paradigm defines wisdom as "expert knowledge that enables us to plan and manage a good life." This definition can be further expanded since there is broad philosophical and scientific agreement that wisdom, like intelligence, is a multifaceted ability. We each develop different forms of wisdom as we age, and each one can compensate for or transcend a weakness or limitation in another.

We can imagine this expansive notion of wisdom as a five-pointed crown that we wear into later life, studded with precious jewels that are continually added each year. The crown and its jewels represent our *reserve*, and consist of all the mental abilities we accumulate over time. The way in which we wear and use the power of this crown represents our *wisdom*. Each point of the crown is a subtype of reserve and wisdom based on the five cited strengths and can be labeled as *savant, sage, curator, creator,* and *seer*. These forms of wisdom apply to every aging person regardless of life circumstances, including those in the ninth stage. Each one is supported by changes in brain activity that enable us to grow and develop new abilities, even in the face of age-related declines in other areas of brain function. They are expressed through unique roles or identities in late life that strengthen with aging and bring greater resilience, purpose, and creativity.

Savant

Even at ninety-four years of age, Mary was faithful to her two Sunday rituals: Catholic Mass in the morning and family dinner in the evening. Her son-in-law Greg would escort her to church and then afterward turn her over to her daughter Victoria for several hours of cooking. Mary's secret was a simple culinary trinity of olive oil, garlic, and a little wine that infused her famous tomato sauce, meatballs, and lasagna. Her grandson would bring over the meats for Mary to chop, grind, and blend into her meatballs; these included pork, veal, steak, and sometimes her special ingredient—pig's knuckles. All her specialty dishes were made from scratch and without written recipes, passed down to Mary from her mother and grandmother and countless generations of Sicilian matriarchs before them. This Sunday ritual brought strength and purpose to Mary over the years, especially after the catastrophic losses, in succession, of her beloved son, daughter, and husband, Sal. She could always count on her remaining family to come over every Sunday afternoon to prepare dinner, join hands in grace, and then dine together. Everyone had a role but Mary had the knowledge and skill to create dishes so perfectly spiced, blended, and baked as to spoil a comparable meal at any Italian restaurant. Mary was also a master seamstress, knitter, and fashion designer who once had a prestigious fashion award presented to her by First Lady Mamie Eisenhower.

Mary embodies the most common and recognizable form of wisdom, characterized by a lifetime reserve of accumulated knowledge, skills, and expertise and the ability to show, share, and teach it. I call this wise person the *savant*, a term derived from the French verb *savoir*, which means "to know" and often designates someone who possesses a specific extraordinary ability. This "aged superhero" connotation of savant is an attribute that most people attain but fail to recognize or celebrate. To the average person, Mary was not renowned for any special abilities, but in her household she was the repository of the family's most meaningful and powerful skills. Her children and grandchildren were entranced hearing her stories and watching and imitating the movements of her hands—how to chop and blend the tomatoes, crush the right amount of garlic, and sprinkle in just so much basil. The pages of a cookbook provide exact measurements of a dish's ingredients, but Mary provided the motions and the meaning, spread out in her mind like the bustling serpentine pathways of the Sicilian town from where her family came. Her roles as a storyteller, expert seamstress, and master Italian cook deepened and matured with age, binding together Mary's family and friends in awe and celebration. She was the wise person described by Sicilian philosopher Empedocles as "honored by all, adorned with holy diadems and blooming garlands."

The strength of the savant lies in the vast reserve of stored knowledge that underlies daily skills and activities. On an anatomic level, this *brain reserve* is determined by the sheer number, density, and connectivity of neurons. On a higher level, it encompasses our *cognitive reserve*, consisting of our baseline intelligence, skills, and experiences, which we bank year by year as a form of mental insurance that allows us to continue functioning normally despite age-related or pathologic damage to our brain. Although it is true that aging brings progressive loss of this reserve, something remarkable happens in the aging brain to compensate. According to the scaffolding theory of aging and cognition, or STAC for short, developed by cognitive scientists Denise Park and Patricia Reuter-Lorenz, older brains can recruit additional networks like a supportive "scaffolding" to accomplish tasks that younger brains do with more limited areas. This process of off-loading mental tasks to other brain regions, called compensation-related utilization of neural circuits, or CRUNCH, is particularly relevant for high-demand mental activities and for high-performing elders. It is common for one aging hemisphere to recruit the other side in a process called hemispheric asymmetry reduction in older adults, or HAROLD. Whether these other brain regions assist by performing the same brain activities or some other strategy is not clear, but such accommodation is key to maintaining expected levels of cognitive function.

Engaging STAC, CRUNCH, and HAROLD is important for the older brain, but additional factors are needed to account for people who seem immune to cognitive aging and perform at normal or supranormal levels compared to individuals thirty or forty years younger. One study of elite pianists, for example, indicated that they maintained such high levels of music-related performance speed by regular and deliberate practice and immersion in musical activities, even though their general processing speed was slowed, consistent with age effects. A group of individuals in their eighties with perfect memories, called "superagers," appear to have none of the expected loss of brain tissue along with an exceptionally developed part of the brain called the left anterior cingulate cortex, or ACC. The ACC has several functions, including attention, motivation, error detection, and emotional awareness—all key components of multiple subtypes of wisdom. There are likely other genetic and lifestyle factors that help explain the state of these fortunate few.

It is important to consider the role of a savant in the ninth stage, when people are less able to speak or otherwise demonstrate their underlying knowledge and skills. Savant wisdom in this stage is more passive but still powerful, gratifying, and meaningful to such individuals and surrounding family, friends, and community. These savants become icons, witnesses, and repositories notable for their long-term memories, residual abilities, and ultimately for their very presence. I am reminded of an eighty-five-year-old woman named Cora, who was the wife of a prominent pastor. Cora's short-term memory was poor, she had no insight into her deficits, and she was prone to paranoid fits in which she would berate her husband, and refuse to take her pills. It was agony at times for her equally aged husband, who still had an enormously important and influential position in their church community. And yet at church events Cora was a role model of the pastor's wife—dignified, charming, regal in her Sunday best (with hat!), and able to quote just the right Bible verse in the company of parishioners.

Cora was venerated by younger women in the church for her experiences during the civil rights era and for raising five successful children. Members of the community understood in a basic way that Cora had some memory problems, but that didn't change their impression nor did it diminish the power of her presence. Although Cora could not remember the events from a recent day gone by, she felt honored and respected in each moment and this bolstered her own identity and mood. Other families might have easily and understandably hidden away a similarly impaired mother. My friend the pastor would do no such thing, however, despite the grief and burden he felt in the face of his wife's progressive dementia.

Sage

Agatha was an eighty-eight-year-old widow who came to me with a relatively severe depression following a car accident in which she had broken her hip and had a lengthy hospitalization with multiple complications. Beneath her depressed facade, she was an incredibly bright and thoughtful woman who was devoted to her family. She had steered relatives through many calamities in life—a destroyed house in Hurricane Andrew, a failed family business, and the loss of her husband—but was always able to right the ship and move forward. Fortunately, Agatha responded beautifully to psychiatric treatment. One day, I received a call from her son Steven and daughter-in-law Jessica. After twenty-five years of marriage, they had separated due to a major rift and were planning to divorce. They were panicked about what, if anything, to tell Agatha. Given how old-fashioned Agatha seemed to them, they were afraid the news would cause her to have a stroke. I suggested that Agatha was more open-minded than they imagined and would be able to deal with whatever news came her way. They were not convinced and kept putting off talking to her until they realized that she would likely hear about their situation from some other source—which could be even more upsetting for her.

Steven and Jessica finally sat down with Agatha and told her the news. They urged her not to panic and promised that she would still see both of them frequently. Expecting the worst, they were shocked by Agatha's reaction. She listened quietly and then asked them why they were so distraught. She held their hands and counseled them to seek the sort of marital counseling that they had avoided for years. She educated them about her own marital strains and the ways in which she and her husband had managed to stay together and repair their relationship. She urged them to include their children in therapy, insisting that a quick and thoughtless divorce would likely fracture the family she had worked to keep together all these years. Steven and Jessica were dumbstruck but sufficiently chastened, and they followed their matriarch's sage advice.

Agatha's attitude reflected a wisdom that goes above and beyond simply having the age-accumulated knowledge and experience of a savant, but involved the addition of insight, values (e.g., the importance of family unity), and virtues (e.g., courage) that are applied to judgments and problem solving. The term *sage* is an appropriate moniker for this form of wisdom, as it is derived from the Latin action verb *sapere*, which means "to taste" and "to discern." Thus, the sage is more than just a *knower*, but a *doer*; not just an expert, but an active judge, mentor, guide, or coach. The sage takes a stance to break an impasse, advance a cause, or render a necessary judgment. Sages are concerned about finding ways to reconcile conflicts and broaden perspectives, with one foot in the past and the other in the future. "Sage" advice has a basis in lessons learned and offers a solution that is directed to a higher purpose.

It is tempting to view the sage as a fully developed thinker, with optimal powers to manipulate mental ideas and solve problems through logic and deduction. Neurologist Elkhonon Goldberg defines such a wise person as an expert at pattern recognition who has been there, done that, and done it again so many times that it's second nature. He believes that we can turn to a lifetime of successful solutions from our "neural library" and apply them to new challenges. A sage's strength is rooted in such highly developed abstract thinking, but he or she can also transcend such patterns when a solution is not immediately apparent. To do so, a sage can suspend the rules of the game, put aside ideology, and consider the context of a problem and the relationships among different or competing approaches or systems. Psychologist Dr. Gisela Labouvie-Vief has described how our aging cognition is better able to integrate and balance out different and even opposing thoughts and feelings, such as our own desires and values and those of other people or belief systems. The decisions we make, then, are better aimed at a common good.

Our sage Agatha, for example, was schooled in a belief system in which divorce was a sin, but she weighed this perspective against her empathic understanding and care for her son and daughter-in-law, having experienced her own marital trials and tribulations. She also looked at the wider context of her competing values and assigned a greater valence to family unity. Experience had taught her how to tolerate both the ambiguity of her shifting beliefs and the uncertainty of a changing world. Seeing an impasse between her son and daughter-in-law, Agatha used both her moral authority and respected position as the family sage to step in and render judgment. A serious rift was bridged and the family could move forward with a more organized and open process of resolution.

Was there anything in Agatha's aging brain associated with her ability to become a sage? One might imagine that CRUNCH and HAROLD may be relevant, as both describe how the aging brain is able to recruit additional regions to weigh and solve problems— analogous to how Agatha is juggling and integrating various interests and ideas. In addition, the secret sauce to the wisdom of a sage lies in the ability to reconfigure long-held emotions, values, and goals. This development is linked to gaining greater control over emotional responses along with deliberate strategies to seek out more positive and meaningful experiences in the face of a shrinking horizon of life. The aging brain is better able to carry out these tasks because the center for emotional regulation, called the orbitomedial prefrontal cortex, or OMPFC, exercises greater control over the amygdala, the part of the brain that prompts fear responses. Steven and Jessica's respective amygdala interpreted the very idea of their rift as something dangerous to Agatha, and this lit up their brain with fear and anxiety. Agatha's brain responded quite differently, as the circuits in her OMPFC, developed by years of experience dealing with major stresses, were able to suppress most fear responses generated by her amygdala and deliver a more controlled, positive emotional reaction. Her wisdom-in-action capability weighed competing values and goals without being burdened by excessive emotionality.

A sage in the ninth stage is often limited in action, but can nonetheless react to stresses and problems with acceptance and persistent engagement. I would call such people *intuitive supporters* since they remain engaged in a mutually beneficial relationship or activity out of an inherent sense of its relevance and importance. Such a ninth stage sage could be found in a hundred-year-old man named Carlos who lived in the nursing home where I work. Carlos was the patriarch of a family in which two of the daughters barely spoke to each other due to an unresolved financial conflict. Even though Carlos had relatively severe memory impairment and physical disability, he would always light up immensely when his daughters would visit. He was a safe harbor for them to coexist in one another's presence, and he facilitated a harmonious setting with his ever-present smiles and caresses. He seemed aware of their conflict and would often pull both daughters' hands together and show a loving facial expression as if to plead for them to get along. An uninformed eye would not grant much strength or influence to Carlos, but without him I feared the family would fracture permanently.

Curator

Irene Weisberg Zisblatt is not your typical tour guide. For the past fifteen years, she has been part of a unique program called the March of the Living that takes thousands of Jewish high school students from around the world on a weeklong trip to Poland each spring to visit various historical sites relating to the Holocaust. This emotional trip culminates on Holocaust Remembrance Day, when these students and their adult chaperones march through the gates of Auschwitz and hold a daylong ceremony to honor the memories of those killed. Irene marches proudly and steadily every year alongside several dozen students from her hometown in Florida. These students adore Irene, and they surround her, hold her arms and hands, and weep as they walk with her down the uneven paths through Auschwitz.

Irene follows the same pathway she walked as a thirteen-year-old girl in 1944, then a prisoner in the camp, stripped of all possessions and freedoms as well as of her parents and five younger siblings, who were all sent to the gas chamber on the day of their arrival in the camp. With the students in tow, Irene tries to describe the indescribable: how she survived starvation, beatings, experimentation by the evil Dr. Mengele, and a trip to the gas chamber in which she clung to the edges of the door and was thrown aside as it was slammed shut on the overcrowded room, leaving her alive on the ramp. Somehow overlooked in the chaos, she survived by hiding under the eaves of the gas chamber's roof. She listened to the agonizing screams of the people crammed into the gas chambers as the Zyklon B pellets were dropped into the room, and then the silence. A sympathetic member of the Sonderkommando—those prisoners forced to work in the gas chambers—was astonished when he saw Irene alive. He plucked her from her hidden perch and, risking his own life, tossed her into a nearby cattle car being sent to a work camp. After several more months of torturous labor and a death march, Irene was liberated by American troops. For a while she lived in a displaced persons camp with other orphaned Jewish children in postwar Europe, until she was able to make contact with relatives in America who sponsored her immigration. After coming to the United States, Irene met her husband, had two children, and settled into a typical suburban life. Along with her memories, Irene carried with her four small diamonds that her mother had given her as a parting gift, hoping they would help her survive.

In her seventies, Irene wrote a book called *The Fifth Diamond* about her experiences as a Holocaust survivor, and began volunteering with the March of the Living. It was critical for her to serve as both a witness and a guardian for the history of the Holocaust, not only for herself and her family but for younger generations of students. Every life lost in the death camps was precious, and Irene committed herself to spreading their memories and messages of life. By connecting with hundreds of students, she was a living history for them to grasp and understand firsthand. She cared enough about these students to travel with them, hand in hand, and retell the lessons of history.

Irene's wisdom is distinct from the savant and the sage since its essence lies in the empathy, concern, and care for others on both a personal, eyeball-to-eyeball level and on a larger community-wide level. She was more than just an expert and a guide; she was also a caretaker for these students. The term *curator* captures these varied roles, since it refers to someone having care and superintendence over both people and a meaningful project or setting. We typically think of a curator as someone who designs and manages exhibits in a museum, but this is only one meaning of the term. Derived from the Latin word *curare*, "to care," and sounding like the word *cure*, the term suggests hope for a resolution to whatever cause the curator is attached to. It is a form of wisdom that links people, ideals, and activities together for the higher purposes of unity, education, and remembrance. Common roles of the curator include being a caregiver for another person; a steward for a cause, environment, or movement; a counselor for individuals needing extra support or guidance; and a committed philanthropist or volunteer for a civic or other charitable organization.

Grandparents are quintessential curators. They are sometimes direct caregivers for their grandchildren and other times caretakers for the values and skills of the family and community. It was once common for grandparents to live in a multigenerational household, where their influence was absolutely formative in the lives of grandchildren. Grandparents may have both the time and the parental experience to exercise the curator's wisdom without being tangled in parent-child conflicts. They are often employed to teach and transport grandchildren when parents are too busy with work. In some cultures, grandparents teach essential skills, such as cooking, sewing, hunting, fishing, and performing religious or tribal rituals. Sadly, this process seems reversed in the digital age, where young people have greater command over technology and are called upon to teach older generations how to use smartphones, the Internet, and social media. It is grandparents and other curators, however, who can teach the essential value of slow and careful analysis. Speed of performance may seem to rule the day, but the older brain takes its time, reads more between the lines, and has the potential for greater comprehension.

Erik Erikson's adult stage of "generativity" is relevant to the curator who uses his or her wisdom to help teach, mentor, and raise a new generation. Vaillant's curator equivalents are the "guardians" who "take responsibility for the cultural values and riches from which we all benefit, offering their concern beyond specific individuals to their culture as a whole . . . looking to the past to preserve it for the future." The wisdom of the curator both overlaps and diverges from these guardians, however, having an equal focus on caring for larger values (such as Irene's writing a book about her cultural and religious history) but taking a more personal approach at times (as with Irene's one-on-one approach). The wisdom of Vaillant's guardian appreciates "irony and ambiguity and enough perspective not to take sides," like an evenhanded judge, whereas that of the curator is sometimes obligated to take a stand in seeking a more personal sense of resolution or justice (such as Irene's refusal to forgive or forget the crimes of the Nazis).

The wisdom of the curator is grounded in empathy and altruism. Empathy is the ability to experience and imagine the feelings and thoughts of others, and is rooted in the brain's ability to perceive and mimic what we observe in other people, mediated by prewired "mirror neurons." The capacity for empathy can deepen with age as we learn more about how our own feelings and thoughts and those of others work. Aging individuals tend to engage in more altruistic behaviors than do equally empathic younger individuals. Empathy in later life tends to be more thoughtful and selective and less emotional, as there is less activation in regions of the aging brain central to emotional processing. Altruistic activities of a curator—such as volunteering or direct caregiving for others—can be immensely satisfying and healthy in late life.

We also see curators in the ninth stage. On a recent trip to Washington, DC, I found myself standing in the airport terminal and fighting back tears as I watched a long line of aged, wheelchair-bound men and women parade by. Each one had an attendant pushing his or her chair, and many were waving, smiling, and swaying to the big band music that was playing at the gate. Several middle-aged men and women dressed in 1940s-era clothes were jitterbugging to the tunes. I was witnessing one of the extraordinary Honor Flights in which an entirely volunteer group brings World War II and Korean War veterans to the nation's capital for a day of touring the major war memorials and being feted for their service to our country. Most of the World War II veterans are in their early to midnineties and many are well into the ninth stage, but despite both cognitive and physical limitations, they retain a sincere desire to represent their service to younger generations. These ninth stage curators can be seen as cultural icons who have the knowledge, experience, and memories of the savant icon but are intent to show it off and serve as living displays.

Creator

The paintings of Cuban American artist Margarita Cano are known for their vivid colors and symbolism for a lost world. Her work *¡Libertad!*, for example, depicts a beautiful woman in a dreamlike state lying on the yellow planks of a wooden raft, with the curls of her charcoal black hair flowing outward like the rolling sea that surrounds her. She is cradling a luminous white rose and a rosy-cheeked infant against her blood red dress. Sharp-toothed gray sharks ply the undulating waves below the raft and a white dove soars above through the star-studded night sky. A basket of plump orange mangoes, a pineapple, and several brilliant yellow plantains nestle into the folds of her dress. The scene conjures the Madonna as fleeing Cuba, the land of Margarita's birth and the obsession of her sadness. "Once upon an island I was happy," she lamented, "I felt free" until she fled Cuba in 1962. It took thirty years of aging and then retirement for Margarita to find a way to express her nostalgia and emotions through painting, and she continues her art now well into her eighties.

Margarita is certainly a curator of memories from the Cuba of days gone by, but she is also a creator of new ways of reshaping and presenting these memories to younger generations. The wisdom of the creator brings tangible products: an artistic piece; a literary work; a new relationship; or an innovative program, perspective, or pathway. It taps into an inner wellspring of age-inspired motivation, interest, grit, and vision to make changes for the present and craft one's legacy for the future. Creators mix together important elements of the past with present ideas and trends in search of new ways of thinking, showing, and doing. Their wisdom is all about hope, just as Margarita described the overall purpose of her art in a gallery profile: "I will continue my quest in pursuit of a happy closure to this never-ending saga."

Creativity is a lifelong attribute and underlies not just artistic endeavors but also novel approaches to problem solving. It is a difficult skill to measure but it has the potential to bloom with increasing age, evidenced not only in the many artists who continued their craft well into their eighties and nineties but also in the everyday lives of individuals who must find ways to work through the many challenges of aging. More than any other thinker, psychiatrist Gene Cohen was the guru of creativity in late life and emphasized over and over that creativity can grow with age and can be applied to so many different areas, including personal expression, adversity, relationships, and community interactions. In his groundbreaking work *The Creative Age*, he introduced his own Einstein-like formula for creative aging: $C = me^2$, where creative expression (C) is a function of the mass (m) of life experience multiplied against the synergistic interactions of our internal psychological and external social experiences (e^2). The essence of Cohen's approach—the very inspiration for this book—is that we must recognize the great potentials we have *because* of aging and not *in spite* of it, with creativity being one of the most powerful and enduring forces.

Indeed, creativity can increase with age because of several key elements. With life experience, we accumulate facts about multiple situations and familiarity with how to deal with problems. The combination and synergy of this mental reserve is what Cohen called *developmental intelligence*, and it only continues to grow and deepen with time and fuel more complex and creative ways of thinking. After retirement and other role changes we often have more freedom to pursue creative interests. Divergent thinking, in which we generate many different possible solutions, is the key to creativity and can increase in aging brains that have a greater flow of activity among different regions (remember CRUNCH and HAROLD?) and with thinking that is less tethered to reactive emotions and rigid attitudes. The older brain builds a motivational reserve that fires our ambition and grit to pursue novel ways of expressing ideas, resolving problems, and connecting individuals and communities.

Creators often differ from our other four wise selves in that they do not always have to rely solely on knowledge and skills from their past. Consider the aging athlete, hobbyist, humorist, artist, craftsperson, or storyteller who is engaging in completely new activities or creative acts that do not have strong connections to their past. There are absolutely elements of savant, sage, curator, and seer in these individuals, but their true strength lies in thinking and acting differently from before, liberated from their past and willing to take risks for the sake of self-improvement, the good of their family or community, or sheer adventure.

We stereotype aging individuals as being stuck in the past and afraid to explore, but this erroneous perception is defied daily by those who seek out unexpected pursuits, new relationships, encore careers, or simply meaningful and liberated styles of life that are, at their root, creative endeavors. Dramatic examples of this type of creator are the flamboyantly dressed and done-up women featured in Ari Seth Cohen's blogs and books as part of his Advanced Style project, dedicated to "capturing the sartorial savvy of the senior set." These aging creators boldly walk the streets of New York City and other locales, wearing dramatically designed dresses, coats, and hats with luminous colors and adornments, all matched with eye-catching jewelry, purses, and glasses. The beauty and celebratory vim of these aging women have caught the attention of the fashion industry, not to mention all who pass them by on the street. You can't miss them in their portrayal of the strengths of aging.

Creators also exist in the ninth stage, but they may need help to unleash forces that reflect intact sensory abilities and that do not rely upon perfect cognition. American artist Hilda Gorenstein, known as Hilgos, was a renowned painter and sculptor whose works in oil and watercolor are in collections around the world. As she developed Alzheimer's disease in her late eighties, Hilgos stopped painting and withdrew into herself. As an experiment, students from the Art Institute of Chicago began working with her to start painting again, and her previous artistry and personality began to reemerge. One day after completing a particularly beautiful watercolor, Hilgos turned to her adoring students and informed them that "I remember better when I paint." This statement inspired her daughter, Berna Huebner, to write a book about how art can open the hidden skills and talents of individuals with dementia, and this was later turned into an award-winning documentary film. In some ways, Hilgos became more influential as a creator in the ninth stage, as her expressive watercolors burst stereotypes of individuals with dementia and promoted the benefits of art therapy.

Seer

Roz's losses, in succession, were staggering: her mother, her aunt, her cousin, and then, suddenly, her beloved partner all died over a two-year period of time. She found herself at age sixty-eight bereft of the key relationships that gave her purpose—as a caregiver, best friend, and life companion. She had even given up her teaching career when she and her partner planned to travel abroad during his sabbatical, only to find herself alone and without employment after his untimely passing. Whereas these encounters with death might cause most people to flee from anything related to the end of life, Roz felt differently. She had been a caregiver and felt that although she did everything she could have done, it wasn't enough. The unexpected death of her partner deprived her of the time to prepare for such a drastic life change. She needed a purpose to fill the emotional void and decided to become a volunteer with a local hospice organization. She enrolled in a six-month training course and then began working with a woman suffering from terminal cancer. Each week, the pair had a ritual to visit a different frozen yogurt store after the woman's chemotherapy. When the woman grew too weak to travel, Roz brought the frozen yogurt to her home.

With time, Roz underwent a major shift in her perspective on life, as the losses had taught her the shortcomings of her rational, organized self: "I let go of my intellectual decision making and just let the universe unfold whatever it had in store for me." She became more spiritual, joined a religious community, and began praying and observing rituals. Her belief in God deepened and she felt freer to make plans and choices based less out of obligation and more on a transcendent sense of her life. She reveled in a sense of gratitude for simply being able to get out of bed each day, wiggle her toes, and spend time meditating and taking long walks while listening to audiobooks. Her goal was not to tell anyone what they should be doing, but instead to serve as a model for good behavior. In her most recent assignment, she has tended to a bed-bound woman with severe dementia who cannot speak to her or offer gratitude, but whose only ability, it seems, is to follow this loving volunteer around the room with her eyes.

The wisdom of the seer is embodied in Roz's transcendent attitude toward her own life and the lives of others. She feels less constrained by artificial boundaries of age-expected roles. She feels a deep spiritual bond to a force greater than her own intellectual powers, and this compels her to do good for others and enables her to feel free to make her own meaningful decisions. She is accepting of her path in life and this radiates to others who feel calmed in her presence. The wisdom of the seer is often expressed in a quiet and reserved manner that may inadvertently appear detached or disengaged. Nonetheless, it is almost always inspiring and even transforming for others.

Technically speaking, the term *seer* refers to someone who can envision or even predict the future, or who receives divine knowledge; literally, a "see-er" of things beyond ordinary sight. In this case, the seer does have extraordinary vision and insight, although not for what will be but for what *could* be. By definition, then, the mind-set of the seer is introspective, inquisitive, and spiritual. It can be directed toward inward contemplation or outward communing with others. For example, some seers employ meditation as a way of seeking solitude or tranquility and giving their brain time and space to contemplate challenges and consider responses. Other seers channel their spiritual selves into religious beliefs and practices and find great satisfaction as part of a community. Both kinds of seers demonstrate enhanced physical and mental health as a result of their practices and connections, even living longer lives as a result.

Seer wisdom helps one cope with change and find meaning and purpose in life; this is why we turn to seers for guidance, support, and inspiration. The image most people have of a beloved parent or grandparent who has died is that of a seer, patiently and peacefully waiting beyond the horizon of life for each of us when we pass on. This perception of the seer as having a connection to forces beyond our seen boundaries is a primal and powerful element of aging. When young people cast their admiring and yearning eyes upon the seer as a guide and support, the experience can fill them with confidence and a deep sense of purpose. Seers themselves do not typically fear death because they have a sense of closeness to a force that embraces their life, along with a sense of closure for the tasks of life that precede the anticipated ending. Gerontologist

Lars Tornstam coined the term *gerotranscendence* to describe this shift in perspective from a more "materialistic and rational perspective" to a more "cosmic and transcendent one."

Even in the ninth stage, the power and influence of the seer is not diminished. I once met the rebbe (spiritual leader) of a close-knit group of Hasidic Jews, who, despite his physical and mental infirmity, was so revered by his followers that his very presence was transformative for those who encountered him. He was not able to lead prayers or deliver sermons as he once did, but he still remembered the motions and the wordless tunes that are the foundation of so many rituals. He could still place his hands on a supplicant's head and emote a blessing, leaving the person nearly ecstatic, because it was such an overlearned behavior programmed into his muscles as much as into his memories. At his *tisch* (table) on the Sabbath, the rebbe could still remember how to make a blessing on the challah bread and then divide it into morsels that his thronging devotees would grab. In this and other similar situations, the ninth stage seer becomes a living relic with a powerful, residual presence that can inspire and give one a feeling of closeness to a divine force. In many major religions throughout history, the term *relics* referred to the physical remains or personal property of a saint or other holy person that are preserved and displayed for devotees. The fortunate ninth stage seer is a living relic who will be revered by individuals who can, in return, provide necessary mutual interactions and care.

Wearing the Crown

Each form of wisdom has corresponding verbs that represent their mutual interactions with others, especially younger generations: the savant *learns*, *shows*, and *teaches*; the sage *weighs* and *decides*; the curator *cares* and *connects*; the creator *imagines* and *makes*; and the seer *accepts* and *communes*. These active forms of wisdom are not always evident or present, however, in aging individuals who are excessively self-absorbed, hedonistic, or disconnected from others. For such people, their daily pursuits are more about *doing* something pleasurable in the moment than *being* or *becoming* something meaningful over time, leading to a lack of purpose outside of acts of self-gratification. This approach represents a form of antiwisdom that is increasingly contagious in our solipsistic digital worlds where so many of the images and sounds we see are facades, rants, and entitlements with little regard for the depth of mutual interactions and for the larger community or society and its sacred relics, rites, and rituals. In this world, aging itself is accorded little meaning or value; and so, we find ourselves back to the beginning of my message.

Let's start again, then, and restate the message but with our deeper understanding: aging is a vexing mystery and brings a natural dread and denigration. To get past this blockage, we need a justification for aging that gives us a sense of meaning, hope, and purpose—the "why" of aging. We can find this in the emergent strengths that aging brings, represented in our wide conceptualization of wisdom as summarized in the Crown of Wisdom table. As we see through our potential roles as savant, sage, curator, creator, and seer, this wisdom activates and elevates our strengths, our mutual interactions, and our missions in life, and in turn makes us valued, wanted, and necessary parts of relationships, families, and communities. Our answer here tells us not simply why we *should* age, but why we *must* age!

The Crown of Wisdom

WISDOM	DESCRIPTION	ROLES	NINTH STAGE ROLES
SAVANT	An individual with a noteworthy accumulation of knowledge, skills, and expertise, and the ability to show, share, and teach it	• Expert • Master/specialist • Storyteller/humorist • Genealogist	• Witness • Repository • Icon
SAGE	An individual whose life experience has generated unique insight and judgment and a commitment to values and virtues that are applied to educating and guiding others, as well as helping others with decision making and problem solving	• Mentor • Guide • Coach • Docent • Leader	Intuitive supporter
CURATOR	An individual with a highly developed sense of empathy, concern, and care for other people, creatures, places, or sacred items or rituals, and the commitment to make benevolent connections with them	• Caretaker • Steward • Counselor • Philanthropist • Guardian • Genetic or foster grandparent/ aunt/uncle	Cultural icon
CREATOR	An individual with the motivation, interest, grit, and vision to build and create, and the active working on artistic, creative, self-improving, and legacy-building endeavors	• Creator • Artist • Craftsman • Athlete • Explorer/traveler • Avid hobbyist/ enthusiast	Guided artist, visitor, or explorer
SEER	An individual with a well-developed sense of insight, spirituality, acceptance, and gratitude toward life, and the active expressing and celebration of these sentiments, in solitude or communing with others who share them	• Volunteer • Counselor • Congregant • Lay clergy • Spiritual guide or leader	• Spiritual icon or figurehead • Living relic

PART II

Why Survive?

When we talk about old age, each of us is talking about his or her own future. We must ask ourselves if we are willing to settle for mere survival when so much more is possible.

—ROBERT BUTLER, *Why Survive? Being Old in America*

Chapter 3

Age Points

THE SEASON BEGAN like every previous year, with heavy snowfall in the mountains each night and early treks to the slopes in the morning. My in-laws Fred and Marlene were like giddy seventy-year-old teenagers on those days, swaggering through the ski lodge, leaping on the chairlifts and then careening down the runs. Friends cajoled and sometimes dared them to try higher and steeper black diamond runs, and they often complied, eager for both the camaraderie and the gut-satisfying sense of control over their body and the white face of the hill. For the past few years it had been retirement heaven for Fred and Marlene and their close circle of friends in Colorado. The only recent glitch had been a bad virus Fred suffered in the early winter, but he passed it off as a nagging cold and had mostly recovered by the time the ski season was in full gear.

But the year abruptly turned in a different direction one morning as Fred was carving his way down the undulating slopes and rises of his favorite run, a beauty called Claimjumper. As he rocketed across one of the final hills with his eyes eagerly searching for the approaching chalet, his left ski hit an unseen patch of ice, scratched out of control, and then twisted abruptly and unnaturally out of rhythm. Fred face-planted on a shelf of snow and then tumbled violently for a few seconds until he plowed into a drift. From the crest of the slope, Marlene saw an explosion of white powder and heard staccato thuds as Fred's body thrashed about. She skidded up behind him in a panicked state, but quickly calmed when she saw him sit up and brush off the snow. He slowly looked up and laughed: he was okay! This reassured Marlene and gave her license to curse him out for being so reckless. As they slowly made their way back down the hill and into the warmth of the chalet, they realized that the fall might have been the result and not the cause of something deeper. Fred had felt winded before the fall and now felt worse. As the day wore on he felt increasingly exhausted, to the point where it was difficult for him to even lift one leg in front of the other. He tried to brush it off, thinking that maybe his virus was back, or perhaps the altitude was bothering him, but Marlene wasn't buying either. A visit to the doctor the next day revealed no physical trauma—no bruises, broken ribs, or even red snow burns on his nose or cheeks that had plowed a path down the icy patch. But he was so pale, and Marlene insisted that the doctor take a closer look. To humor her he drew some blood, and they left for the day with Fred feeling reassured and Marlene apprehensive.

The next day the doctor called with some bad news. Fred's blood counts were all perilously low, with every component of his blood—corpuscles, platelets, and white cells—dangling well below a danger zone where there was great risk of infection, bleeding, and ischemia. Fred needed to be seen in the nearby clinic in Frisco immediately, which led within days to a hematologist in Denver. A slew of tests, including the first of what would be many bone marrow biopsies, revealed a grave-sounding diagnosis: leukemia. For Marlene, the news hit her like a terrible spill she had taken down the slope her first year skiing—tumbling and flailing painfully out of control and feeling battered and bewildered afterward.

Fred's initial reaction was silence and morbid shock, and it triggered immediate memories of the blood disease that had killed his middle-aged mother many decades before—far too early in both of their lives. Surprisingly, the doctor was less concerned and he explained his chipper demeanor: Fred had a form of the blood disease known as hairy cell leukemia, a less common but eminently manageable condition that often responded to initial treatment with long-term remission. This clarification brought Fred and Marlene a sigh of relief but the shock was still there, and they understood intuitively that the trajectory of their lives had taken a major deviation. Nothing would ever be quite the same.

A New Question of Why

We face challenges and struggles most days of our lives. Sometimes we take them in stride and have well-worn pathways to address them, and sometimes they push us off our game. In both cases, we typically take note of the stress, pivot, and move on. For example, Fred and Marlene had both fallen before, been sick before, and faced medical issues before. In fact, they had been through lots of stressful situations in the past and always coped well. In this case, however, there were new and unexpected elements. Marlene had a fleeting thought that Fred was seriously injured or even killed by his fall. In an instant, she ran through a deck of cards in her mind that contained most of her existential worries: Fred's being disabled and her needing to be his caregiver, the end of skiing and biking, the end of her halcyon life in Colorado, and the end of her life with Fred if he died. In previous contemplations of these inevitable scenarios, she didn't have a vision of getting beyond them. She conflated them with the end of her own life. Fred's diagnosis splayed these cards in front of her, and she was overwhelmed with the worry that her doomsday was beginning. Fred did not brood over this scenario as Marlene did, but his diagnosis connected the very raw loss of his mother with fears of his own mortality. It was as if a phantasm had risen from the grave and grabbed his heel as he was zooming down the hill, pulling him facedown in his exuberance and pride.

Their shock was compounded in short order by the sudden illness and death of a woman in their close circle from leukemia, the divorce of a couple they had known for years, and the onset of Alzheimer's disease in another lifelong friend. In a matter of months, their world seemed to be tipping over into the old age they had feared for so long. They had been enjoying aging up until this point, guided by a clear mission that answered their personal question of why age. Now, a new and more insidious question appeared: *Why survive?* In the face of a direct threat to the most cherished aspects of an aging lifestyle, what is the point to living in the face of such daunting struggles? How does one find a way to navigate challenges that seem insurmountable? Where is the meaning and joy in it?

Age Points

One way to frame our experiences and response to adversity is through a concept I am calling an *age point*. An age point is a period of time in which an event or situation prompts a significant disruption in our initial ability to understand and cope with it. It exposes a gap between the challenges or demands of a life event and our existing strengths, values, skills, and connections. An age point might begin with a moment of crisis, trauma, or even terror, and causes us to feel temporarily stunned or paralyzed, and uncertain about what to do. We may want and need to respond, but we don't know what will be effective to resolve the situation and regain our balance. Even though an age point exposes a weakness, it is also loaded with the potential for tremendous growth if we can navigate the two sides of the gulf and create a bridge to link them together. Resolving an age point makes us into more developed and capable aging adults. The greatest challenge of an age point is having to give up previous notions, identities, and ways of doing things in the service of a solution.

Age points fall into four distinct stages:

1. **Event:** The circumstances strong enough to prompt an age point
2. **Suspension:** The period of profound uncertainty and paralysis
3. **Reckoning:** The intellectual, emotional, and behavioral process of weighing, confronting, and attempting to reconcile the gaps between what we have and what we need
4. **Resolution:** A new way of looking, thinking, feeling, and doing that bridges the gap and allows us to regain our balance and move forward

An age point can take days, months, or even years to unfold and resolve, and the outcome is not necessarily a positive one. Fortunately, we can prepare for age points and actively guide the process to something positive even if we cannot imagine what that may be. The key is to optimize one's reserve and wisdom ahead of time and develop our age-conferred strengths of resilience and creativity. Let's explore the stages of age points in more detail.

Event: The nature of the event or situation that triggers an age point is less important than how it is experienced and interpreted. Common triggers include a major injury or illness in oneself or a loved one; a major life stress, such as a divorce or financial setback; a failure of a major task or project; a significant role shift, such as due to retirement; and even a positive milestone, such as a major birthday or the wedding of a child. Not every trigger has to constitute a clear crisis or trauma, but it must have sufficient emotional and intellectual impact to disrupt a person's underlying script. Life events are more likely to trigger age points in individuals who have brittle supportive relationships (e.g., a loveless marriage), rigid beliefs (e.g., absolute opposition to mental health care), or singular attachments (e.g., reliance on one adult child for all needs).

Suspension: The Greek philosophers believed that the suspension of judgment and commitment (what in Greek they called *epoché*, pronounced "eh-poh-kay´") provided an ideal state of mind in which to examine the world. A later school of philosophy called phenomenology believed that this suspension provided a method of experiencing things more freely and less influenced by all the assumptions that color our perceptions. Thus, it is a state of mind suspended from our normal script. As an age point unfolds, this "suspension" is an ideal term to describe the deep state of uncertainty and confusion that occurs when our established assumptions or scripts cannot understand and process our current circumstances. We might liken this to the state of shock that occurs during a trauma, but without the depth of physical and emotional detachment. The suspension can be a positive state when we put aside previous assumptions that are prejudiced and limiting, and begin to think in broader and more creative ways. When negative, however, the suspension of the age point is a muddled state of mind with significant emotional tension that makes decision making difficult. We may lose our sense of meaning in the world, leaving us feeling shattered and vulnerable. Individuals who are emotionally overwhelmed by the suspension may lapse into deep anxiety or depression, have severe panic attacks, or even succumb to transient moments of psychosis in which they lose touch with reality.

Reckoning: The term *reckoning* refers to the act of estimating the amount or cost of something as well as facing a day of judgment when a debt, verdict, or decision is called. During age points, the process of reckoning forces us to examine our shortcomings and acknowledge that there is a problem. We must estimate the cost of reconsidering certain beliefs, relationships, or behaviors and face moments of change. We begin such reckoning from a previous position of strength that we relied upon, trusted to be our guide, and are reluctant to give up. By the definition of an age point, however, this position is not working. One can certainly try to avoid such reckoning, but there is great risk of perpetual suspension in which we regress into rigid and dysfunctional patterns of thought or behavior.

During the stage of reckoning, we begin to question our beliefs and our abilities. We may have a crisis of faith. It is painful to realize that trusted things have failed us in some way. We begin to enumerate what's not working and consider alternatives. We calculate the process and price of making changes. We wonder how others might respond to our tribulations, and conjure up images and voices of parents, grandparents, and other authority figures in our lives. By its very nature, the process of reckoning might be the longest part of the age point, since we have to weigh whether we really want to make changes, imagine all the permutations, and allow both our emotions and our intellect to sit with each consideration and decide whether it feels right and is worth pursuing. As we begin to make decisions and mobilize our energy, we engage in self-monitoring of our actions and strategies to gauge whether they are meeting our goals, and if not, we correct course.

Resolution: A resolution to an age point is composed of a new set of beliefs and behaviors that close the gaps between the individual's abilities and the demands of the situation that triggered the age point in the first place. Ideally, a new person arises from the age point with a more flexible and functional approach and a greater sense of well-being. Pathologic components of the age point, such as depression, anxiety, or substance use, should be improved if not resolved. The resolution may also reflect a failure of development and growth, due to resistance or regression. We may refuse to make changes or give up long-held beliefs or behaviors, and instead create a protective but limited and fragile bubble around us or regress into behaviors that provide immediate gratification but stunt our growth.

☞

On the other side of their age point, in the resolution stage, Fred and Marlene have little memory of their visceral reactions to Fred's illness. The fears, sadness, anger, and confusion of the suspension have receded and are difficult to conjure. During the period of reckoning, they began to question how they could maintain their previous lifestyle. They returned to skiing for a while, but began to focus more on the downside as a way to rationalize giving it up: achy knees, fear of injury, and disdain for the growing crowds on the slopes. Their previous avoidance and skepticism of doctors had to be reconsidered since Fred's condition was a matter of life or death and they had no choice but to rely on them. Marlene had her battles with the doctors and nurses and had to carefully decide when to resist and demand and when to acquiesce. Both Fred and Marlene had to learn to trust a much wider circle of people.

As this reckoning unfolded, each wore his or her crown of wisdom well. Marlene became Fred's sage, weighing each medical fact and figure presented to her by the doctors, asking question after question, and then advising Fred what he should do. Her role as a savant for organization kicked in, since she had to plan their calendar around his medical care and ultimately organize regular trips to the National Institutes of Health to enable Fred to receive experimental treatment. Fred emerged as a seer, finding acceptance and even some serenity in knowing that somehow everything would work out. "The situation made me stronger because I didn't have a choice," he recalled. "I had to do what I had to do. Eventually, I was able to look to others and get strength from them." This was a huge change for a fiercely independent man who was used to running the entire show.

The resolution followed from their wisdom and adaptation. They sought out the best care they could find and then trusted the doctor to work his magic—which he did, to a complete remission after four lengthy attempts. They moved from a community up in the mountains down to the city of Denver and started a new life without skiing and hiking, but with many other meaningful pursuits. Fred retired from the pressure of his accounting practice. He is no longer preoccupied with work and is able to spend more time with friends and family in a relaxed and free-flowing manner. Marlene was clear about the change: "I grew up a lot in the last six years." She adjusted her expectations of what she could do in life and found greater acceptance of her limitations. Many years ago, she once told me that I ought to "shoot her" if things got really bad in her old age. I don't see that Marlene anymore: she is able to adapt. I am confident that Fred and Marlene will be able to face the changes ahead with newfound strengths, and it was the age point surrounding Fred's illness that made all the difference.

What Do Age Points Give Us?

Age points illustrate the transitions we make in life, and can occur at any time and under many circumstances. Although they might occur within a major stage or change of life, such as midlife, menopause, or retirement, they also allow us to examine our own experiences in the moment, untethered from any developmental milestones or scheme. Age points can even apply to individuals in the ninth stage, who are otherwise effectively left out of all current life cycle theories and models.

CB

When I first met Arturo and Flavia, I met the whole family. They came to my office accompanied by their two sons and daughters-in-law in person, and their daughter joined via phone. Arturo's brother came, since he was a physician and wanted to offer his thoughts. Flavia's sister and housekeeper also attended. My assistant had already circulated through the crowded room and offered bottles of water and small cups of Cuban coffee, and by the time I entered it sounded like a raucous family reunion, fueled in part by potent jolts of caffeine. In my past lives as a doctor in Boston and Minneapolis, such a scene would have been overwhelming, but this was Miami and it was just another Monday morning clinic. Arturo and Flavia's large group, all originally from Venezuela, were like many of the Cuban and South American families, Christian and Jewish alike, who come to my memory center as *la familia enterra* or *die gantze mishpocha*—the whole family—seeking my counsel and wanting to give input and provide support from every angle.

Arturo spoke first. He was seeking a second opinion because his wife had recently been diagnosed with Alzheimer's disease by a local neurologist, but he didn't believe it. He argued that the memory changes reported by his children and sister-in-law were exaggerated. Flavia had always been somewhat absent-minded, he argued, and this accounted for most of the negative assessments, including that of the neurologist who "really didn't know her." Flavia's provisional diagnosis, however, had thrown him into a deep state of anxiety, and he reported difficulty sleeping and eating. Because he ran a successful import-export company, which took him out of the country for long trips, he urgently needed to know that Flavia would be okay.

I turned to Flavia, who was sitting quietly next to her husband with an anxious smile on her face. She was impeccably made up and beautifully dressed, as if she were attending a dinner party and not on a visit to the doctor. She spoke to me in English with frequent lapses into Spanish when she couldn't come up with the right word. She was aware of her family's concerns, but didn't see the same problems with her memory. As she spoke, she often would pause to search for a word, and look to her husband for a hint. "You, *you* have to tell him!" he bellowed at her each time.

Her daughter Sofia suddenly broke in over the phone, and implored me to take their concerns seriously in contrast to what their father was saying. Flavia's sister Patricia started crying and nodding her head in agreement as she listened, and then interrupted to add that their mother had suffered from Alzheimer's disease and she was seeing the exact same symptoms in Flavia. Arturo's brother spoke up next, expressing exasperation at the previous doctor's hasty diagnosis and insisting that a full workup had not been conducted. The two sons listened and seemed to be torn between their father's and sister's differing opinions. Their questions focused on how I could help them find more resources for their parents. When they finished speaking, all eyes turned toward me.

Up to that point, the meeting had been a little bit like the 1950 Japanese film *Rashomon*, where a single event gets described from multiple contradictory angles. It was clear that the couple was facing a major age point, and in the throes of this crisis they were tasking me to guide them through to the other side. But I had to somehow find a way to harmonize the disparate voices into a common pitch. Clearly, the tentative diagnosis of Alzheimer's had thrown Arturo into the suspension of an age point, causing him to be stunned, deeply anxious, and uncertain about where to turn. He resisted the diagnosis and tried repeatedly to explain away Flavia's symptoms. He was stuck at that point, lacking the knowledge to make further conclusions and preoccupied with suppressing his anxiety. Flavia was equally uncertain and frustrated, wanting to please both her husband and her sister at the same time that she was clearly struggling with increasing short-term memory deficits.

Sometimes the best approach during the suspension is to get people back to their safe spots. Arturo needed a logical process of inquiry and some hope, and Flavia needed some reassurance and family harmony. I knew I could help here but that the patch would only be temporary. Still, I hoped it would give the whole family more time to absorb the changes and marshal resources. I began by thanking all of them for coming and acknowledging the power of their family unity. I praised Arturo for his fierce dedication to Flavia and stated my commitment to finding a solution. I gave them a vision of a comprehensive assessment and treatment plan that transcended the diagnosis; in other words, we would work together no matter what was revealed. Everyone could feel as if he or she was actively working on a solution, even without knowing the exact diagnosis. After a lengthy explanation of the necessary workup, including brain scans and cognitive testing, I listened to the family's concerns and answered their questions. Even in the midst of this age point, Arturo and Flavia were able to have a moment of hope.

Age points do not unfold in linear patterns. There is much seesawing between the gaps of the situation before strengths can begin to emerge and create a solution. Such was the case with Arturo and Flavia, and they struggled for some time. Flavia was not fully aware of her short-term memory loss, but was noticeably frustrated, confused, and resistant to help. She insisted on taking her own medications but made regular mistakes that resulted in several medical crises, including sky-high blood pressure when she forgot to take her medication and a fainting spell when she took too much.

Arturo was acutely aware that Flavia's memory had declined, but he detested and resisted the idea that she had Alzheimer's disease, to the point of full denial. Out of frustration and avoidance, he began taking long business trips out of the country for weeks on end. He began drinking more alcohol, sleeping less, and driving himself to expand his business, as if that would somehow compensate for Flavia's losses. Every discussion with his children became an argument. He accused Flavia's sister of creating the whole situation in the first place and stopped talking to her. His brother tried to intervene, but Arturo simply couldn't discuss the inevitable diagnosis. Even as his suspicions grew, however, he avoided setting up a follow-up appointment until his sons forced the issue.

When we met to review the test results, I suggested gently that everything pointed toward a likely diagnosis of Alzheimer's disease. Arturo wanted to know what Flavia's PET scan showed, and I told him it was positive, meaning that it showed evidence of significant amounts of the toxic beta-amyloid protein in her brain. He looked at me in disbelief, and then the emotional dam broke. He began sobbing uncontrollably, as if the entire weight of evidence had finally sunk in. It was a painful, agonizing moment for everyone in the room, but provided the necessary emotional release to unblock Arturo's avoidance and endless, rigid reckoning. He was ready to move forward.

Navigating the Age Point

In this case, Arturo and Flavia were surrounded by supportive family and doctors who could stand by during the age point and help craft a solution. Some people are not so fortunate, and end up spinning and spinning in the suspension without being able to face reality. To relieve such emotional turmoil, these stuck individuals often end up retreating into depression, anxiety, substance abuse, compulsive behaviors, or rigid lifestyles. These responses are only partially helpful as they replace one form of distress with another that initially feels better but stunts personal growth and carries a risk for further crises and paralysis.

Other people can move beyond the suspension and into a period of reckoning, but they cannot reconcile opposing perspectives or ideologies and stretch their intellect beyond a very narrow and fixed worldview. As a result, they abandon any meaningful discussion or consideration of their circumstances and plunge or retreat into false beliefs, ideologies, estrangements, or contradictory relationships. Such aging brings a fierce circling of the wagons and an unhealthy narcissism. Think of an aging dictator who cannot accept the possibility of relinquishing power and maintains an oppressive and sclerotic regime at any cost. On a smaller scale, these are aging individuals who cut themselves off from family members who refuse to follow their dictates or who live lifestyles they find unacceptable. There is simply no compromise, but this rejectionist approach carries great risk of further impasses and crises.

There are also individuals who bail out of the reckoning stage by refusing to do anything: they *disengage*. They may do this because they don't believe that they have the mental or physical ability to change. They might be frightened of the consequences. They might be exhausted or preoccupied by some other stressor. Or they might not actually have the resources to effect change because they are in the ninth stage. We used to believe that disengagement was a natural part of aging, and so we didn't expect people to change and we stereotyped them as rigid and impaired (we sometimes still do!). There is simply no significant research to support such a theory, and we know instead that aging often brings the opposite—*engagement* across a wide swath of issues and activities. Nonetheless, we should view a disengaged aging person as someone who is struggling with the possibility of change and still retains the capacity to move forward, even if he or she doesn't believe it.

Up until his emotional release, Arturo was trying to find an easy out of the reckoning phase. He was faced with trying to reconcile his enduring belief in Flavia as a cognitively intact, full partner in their marriage, with an image of her as diminished and dependent. In clinging to the former belief, he began to disengage with anyone who suggested otherwise. He contemplated a complete rejection of all her doctors and instead began researching several radical and wholly unproven therapies that promised an instant cure. Flavia was having a difficult time herself, since her insight into her memory changes was poor and getting worse, and she resented anyone's labeling her as impaired and treating her like a child. She also began to disengage from friends and relatives. How was it possible to breach this impasse with them?

Getting beyond the point of reckoning and into the resolution stage of an age point requires two strengths that may seem to be moving in opposite directions. On the one hand, people need to grab on to their anchors of reserve, represented by beliefs, skills, memories, and relationships that provide stability and consistency. On the other hand, they need to follow the path suggested by French author Marie de Hennezel to "let go of our past, become reconciled with ourselves, and accept that we will be diminished in one respect in order to grow in another." Accomplishing both tasks seems contradictory, but is necessary and has a cabinet of allies in our five wise selves. The savant brings the necessary skills, while the sage forges a compromise; the curator engages with the desired customs and communities, while the creator crafts new ways to think and act. Finally, the seer harmonizes the various perspectives into a vision of life that enables us to fully accept and find meaning in the resolution.

Arturo could no longer push away the reality of Flavia's illness. In his catharsis during our meeting, he bent but didn't break by leaning on his core strengths: his street smarts and business acumen, his family connections, and his deep and abiding love for Flavia. He also let go of the impediments to change. Within a few weeks of our meeting, he took several radical steps that seemed unlikely the month before—but now flowed easily. He turned over his business to his sons and assumed an advisory capacity. He decided to manage Flavia's care with the same energy and creativity that he had managed his business. He reengaged with his entire family and began directing them in ways to be most useful. It was a stunning turn of events, but the seeds of it were always present and it took the rocky ride of the age point to break them down and grow them. The end of the age point revealed two more age-emergent strengths that pushed it along: resilience in the face of stress, and a deep sense of purpose.

Chapter 4

Being Resilient, Pursuing Purpose

IT WAS TIME, I thought, to call in hospice. Muriel seemed to be at the end of her eighty-year-old road. She had suffered from excruciating back and leg pain for the past four years, and from a sad bevy of maladies for several decades prior to that. Now she was doped up on morphine and delirious from pancreatitis likely caused by excess use of said morphine. She lay in her hospital bed and stared at the wall, contorted by pains in her gut from the leaking digestive enzymes and from muscle spasms in her back from the inflamed connective tissue that ran up and down her spine and around the rods and screws that held it all in place. A plastic drainage tube from her stomach spiraled up and out of her nose and into a suction bottle next to the bed to help reduce the persistent nausea and vomiting. Her kidneys were failing and her intestines—a hodgepodge of cut-up and reconnected loops from previous surgeries—were paralyzed without any sustenance to squeeze. She looked pale and gaunt from having shed 30 pounds in the past month.

Muriel's body and brain were under massive assault, billowed and battered from every angle by searing pain, immobility, and depression. Still she tried to fight back. The adrenal glands sitting atop her kidneys were pumping out streams of stress hormones to rev up her metabolism and quiet the storm triggered by the aching, inflamed tissues in her belly and back. Control centers in her brain were trying to bear the load and restore some balance to her system. In the short run, Muriel's body could keep things afloat, but with time her illnesses, medications, and protective responses would further weaken her and begin damaging vital brain cells and circuits. She was severely ill and approaching a point of no return.

I see aging individuals like Muriel every day who are facing daunting stresses to both body and mind. Sometimes, the stresses are wholly medical crises, as with Muriel; other times, they begin as financial or social blows and then affect everything else. Shirley, for example, described a cascade of events that began when she was seventy-two years old with a major financial crisis and led to the loss of her car and home, a severe depression, and then an addiction to prescription drugs. Sometimes they are forces of nature that affect the entire community, such as Hurricane Katrina in 2005, in which thousands of older individuals lost their homes, their social supports, and in too many cases, their lives. Major stresses can be sudden or insidious personal affronts, betrayals, or losses, such as with seventy-five-year-old Geoffrey, who discovered that his son was siphoning excess funds from his bank account, or sixty-eight-year-old Sylvia, whose husband developed pancreatic cancer and died within four months. In both cases, their grief was compounded by the additional burden of having to disentangle complex finances and figure out who to trust for support. Geoffrey was distraught and lapsed into an old gambling addiction, whereas Sylvia developed a painful inflammatory condition and panic attacks. Each of these situations raises our key question: Why survive the stresses of aging when hope for anything better seems lost?

Aging appears to be a major liability in the face of such stresses, increasing the risk of severe and permanent illness, pain, and disability, if not death. It's a lesson learned from studying the impact of stress on the aging brain and body, which become more vulnerable to injury and less responsive during recovery. It's also a lesson learned in most major natural or human-made disasters, when it's more difficult for older individuals to safely hunker down or outrun the danger because of lesser physical, social, and financial resources. Once it is upon them, they bear the load more severely than do the young and are more prone to dehydration, injury, and death. Even when they survive, there is a heightened risk for all sorts of mental and physical maladies and deprivations that can leave them languishing for sufficient help or even threatened with abandonment. Under these clouds, can aging bring any light?

When We Bend in Old Age, Why Don't We Break?

In the days leading up to Hurricane Katrina's assault on the Gulf Coast of the United States in late August 2005, the warnings were stark but not always heeded. Too many older residents in the small coastal towns along the beaches, bays, and bayous of Louisiana and Mississippi thought they could withstand the storm, buoyed in part from memories of having survived Hurricane Camille in 1969 and more recent close calls with Hurricanes Ivan and Dennis. Few imagined the direct gut-punch that would hit, bringing with it historic 20- to 30-foot storm surges that accompanied the furious winds and wiped away countless homes and businesses right down to their concrete slabs. Thousands of older residents who stayed behind were left injured and homeless but alive, and there was a small but significant group of less fortunate ones who were killed outright by the storm or died shortly thereafter from their injuries.

In her account of the storm's fury in the small Mississippi coastal town of Bay St. Louis, author and resident Ellis Anderson recounts the tales of some of these older survivors who emerged from the storm shaken and shell-shocked like everyone else, but ready to rebuild. From their refuges in cars, rickety remnants of homes, and other makeshift shelters, these aging residents were part of the backbone of the recovery. Like everyone in the path of the storm, they faced the same losses, traumas, and forced relocations. In some ways, they had more to lose, given their deep roots in the historical neighborhoods that were torn apart or washed away in the storm. We know that they represented a disproportionate number of the physically injured and dead. Yet psychologically, these aged residents did not fare any worse, and in many cases, they coped better than others. Their secret lay in the strength of resilience that was forged and developed through aging.

Resilience refers to the ability to cope with adversity and regain one's footing or balance afterward. From the body's perspective, it's a return to homeostasis, in which stress-induced alterations in heart rate, muscle tension, hormones, neurotransmitter release, and other protective mechanisms begin to ebb and return to normal. On the level of the person, resilience involves being able to acknowledge and then respond to surrounding stress or trauma in ways that allow a return to previous psychological functioning. Sometimes, the traumatic experiences are so severe that they return unannounced or in response to seemingly innocuous triggers. Sufferers of post-traumatic stress disorder, or PTSD, for example, relive the trauma through intrusive memories, or flashbacks, accompanied by emotional or behavioral symptoms that mimic the body's and brain's reactions as if actual danger is crashing down. In most studies of PTSD, aging is a neutral factor, neither causative nor particularly protective. A deeper dive into the lives of survivors, however, shows how resilience can be powered by aging.

In their study of older survivors of Hurricane Katrina five years after the storm, social workers Susan Hrostowski and Timothy Rehner focused on a highly resilient sample to learn how aging made a difference. Many of their findings support my own impressions, from working with hundreds of aging individuals, that our five forms of wisdom become the first and most critical stabilizing elements. The knowledge and expertise of the savant, gained from decades of facing adversity, gives us a range of survival skills and a feeling of competence to face the challenges in front of us. The older storm-battered survivors of Katrina, for example, had been through the Great Depression and World War II and were less reactive to the losses of such services as cell phones, computers, and the Internet, which they viewed more as luxuries than necessities. They knew firsthand how to be resourceful in the face of scarce resources.

The decision-making skills of the sage enable us to allocate resources to ourselves and others in ways that are most fair and practical. Ellis Anderson tells a story of a grandfather who chose to live in his car on her property in the aftermath of the storm so as to care for a beloved dog that would otherwise be too disruptive in the house where the rest of his family was sheltering. Such decision making can provide a sense of involvement and benevolent control over an otherwise chaotic setting. The empathy and altruism of the curator helps to remind others of the core values of the community, and sets up role models, such as the two elderly brothers in Anderson's account who used their generator to set up a free electrical charging station in the town. Such actions bring curators into new caring relationships and leave them feeling useful and wanted by the community.

The curiosity and grit of the creator is key to devising workarounds and other solutions in the face of adversity, such as the two older landlords from one of Anderson's stories who saved themselves and a neighbor in the flooded streets of New Orleans by devising an evacuation spot with a lean-to jerry-rigged out of tarps and an observation post made from scrap lumber. The actions of the creator can not only guarantee survival but also bring an important sense of one's ability to achieve and succeed. The seer is able to see beyond the chaos and threats of major stresses and find moments of acceptance and hope, such as the ninety-year-old disabled woman who took refuge in Anderson's house during the storm and was able to remain calm, accept the care she needed and express humor and gratitude in response. Even in her debilitated state, she was an inspiring role model in the face of adversity.

In each of these descriptions, it is clear how wisdom comes to serve an even broader role when activated by stress and trauma. True to its definition, it provides the strengths we need to manage the challenges at hand. At the same time, it brings us closer to others and others closer to us in a mutual bonding across generations and other imagined boundaries. This wisdom-in-action makes us feel needed and essential. Our aging selves do not have to be a burden to others as may have been the case in ancient tribes under siege who needed to fight or run, but can be key repositories of knowledge and know-how, arbiters and advocates of values, voices of hope, and role models of endurance. Resilience based on our wisdom can transform ourselves and others around us, bringing positive emotions and enhanced self-esteem. Mere survival gives way to growth.

In the moment, wisdom will serve us quite well during and after times of stress and trauma. It is one of the major elements in the formula that determines our resilience. Trying to understand or even predict the eventual outcomes of a major stress on any given aging individual will, however, require a much deeper exploration of the origins and development of this wisdom as it unfolds over our lifetime. It will show us a more complete analysis of how far a specific person can bend under stress without breaking—like the bowing and twisting trunk of a palm tree in a hurricane's winds—flexible and sturdy up to a point until it either snaps or is lifted out by its failing roots.

CR

In the months leading up to her hospitalization, Muriel was wavering between feeling just good enough to function and total collapse. She had already endured years of physical ailments, and had survived by placing her trust in the hands of chosen doctors. Her state of chronic pain, however, was breaching this approach. She had been given frequent increases in her pain medications and was receiving regular steroid injections up and down her back, but with diminishing relief and even increased pain during and after the procedures. Twice a month she would arrive at the treatment center at four a.m., be prepped for the procedure, undergo general anesthesia, and have a large needle pressed into one of the narrowed and misaligned spaces between her vertebrae. A powerful steroid solution would then be injected. Afterward, her daughter and aide would ferry her torpid body back home, where it would take two days for her to come back to life. She would have a few good days without severe pain, but inevitably it would roar back the same as before.

Each month, between such injections, Muriel would hobble into my office with the aid of her walker and cry out in pain and despair. Both talk therapy and medications failed her, and I had no other remedy to give. Month after month I urged her to come to our specialized pain center for a second opinion, but she clung to her one pain doctor and the incessant injections, hoping that the *next* one would do the trick. Before too long, she was lying in the hospital and bending to the point of near breaking, saved only by the fact that she was in too much pain and mental agony to actually carry out a suicide plan. I pictured in my mind the Muriel

I first met some ten years prior when she brought in her husband, Buddy, to evaluate his failing memory and belligerent behaviors. She was stressed then, too, but had a resolute spirit from having survived so many medical problems and crises, in part by being the supreme caregiver for others. By projecting her care needs onto others, she always had a mission that suppressed any excessive focus on her own physical pain and occasional disability. This approach, unfortunately, was no longer working. Younger Muriel had been a spring who always bounced back, but aged Muriel was more rigid. Young Muriel had the resources to fight her own battles, but aged Muriel needed help from others.

At this juncture, however, we find not only Muriel but all aging selves in a potential dilemma. The equation that determines how we survive as we age in the face of stress is difficult to compute. There are many factors to consider and quantify in terms of their positive or negative influence. Even when we try, the formula can reveal different possibilities depending on how fixed or flexible we may be at that moment, and it changes with time and increasing age. It seems like an overwhelming and ultimately fruitless task, which is why, I believe, we often abandon even trying. Instead, many thoughtful minds find it easier to focus on the clear and salient declines, diseases, and decrepitudes of later life and assume that they will rule the day since the ultimate end is death and not eternal life. We see this fatalism in the assumption that we cannot improve beyond a certain age. This is a common, often unconscious and fundamentally ageist perspective constrained by a narrative and perhaps even an ideology of decline. We can easily project this belief onto Muriel, assuming that the storm surge was coming in and washing away any possibility of a positive outcome. She would bend and then break. Why then, should she try to survive? Was there a force that could provide salvation?

Let's Look Beyond the Moment

We've been looking at Muriel as a model for many aging individuals in a storm of stress *in the moment*. Such terrible and sometimes tragic times drive the most trying of age points, and are the culmination of events that may seem insurmountable. It's important to take a step back, however, and examine the long life that preceded these circumstances to be able to see clearly how the vagaries of aging including its emerging strengths of wisdom can power us through them. We can then see not simply how our aging selves *react* in time, but how we *develop and grow* over time. We see how we are not just *passive* figures in the face of stresses, but *active* agents of change. An overview of Muriel's life cycle is revealing.

Muriel grew up in Yonkers, New York, the daughter of a workaholic American doctor married to her Scottish mother. She was raised in a strict household with an almost fanatical work ethic and zeal for doing the right thing. This environment may have stemmed, in part, from lessons learned from her father's rise from a poor family that had to steal coal off train cars to keep warm in the winter. Muriel met her husband, Buddy, at the age of twenty, when they were both in a wedding party, and their own wedding followed six months later. She raised a son and daughter and maintained a lifetime devotion to her husband, even through the fifteen years of his progressive decline and then death from Alzheimer's disease.

Muriel's life has been shaped by two major roles, as a patient and as a caregiver. Her daughter, Ellyn, reeled off all her mother's major illnesses in succession: breast cancer and a double mastectomy at the age of fifty, irritable bowel syndrome and a history of multiple intestinal surgeries, arthritis, a bleeding ulcer that nearly killed her, chronic back and leg pain, multiple back surgeries, kidney failure, her most recent bout of pancreatitis, and a dependence on opioid pain medications. She has coped with all these illnesses by being a relentless caregiver for others. She worries about everyone but herself and makes everybody's problems her problems. Her greatest pleasure is doing for others, and she does so in a warm, empathic, and determined way without ever complaining and with deep gratitude for everything that comes her way. She has had many small extended families that consider her like a grandmother. She is stubborn in her generosity, always kind and honest, smart, conscientious, and insistent on helping others, sometimes to her own detriment.

When considering Muriel's entire life instead of just a few moments, then, we see a much grander and complete picture. She has built up a whole portfolio of strengths that set the stage for her ability to cope with the stresses of illness and redirect or rechannel her anxiety, pain, and loss of control into caring for others by easing or controlling their painful stresses. She has fulfilled the challenge of Erik Erikson's eighth stage of development (i.e., "old age"), which is to develop a sense of completion, wholeness, and "integrity" instead of feeling despairing or even disgusted over final struggles, missing pieces, or failures. She has acquired the key predictors of aging discovered by psychiatrist George Vaillant in Harvard's decades-long Grant Study of Adult Development, including good relationships with others; a good marriage; a sense of humor about life; a strong focus on friendship; altruistic behaviors; and keen senses of forgiveness, gratitude, and lovingkindness. She has embodied the one key predictor of longevity discovered by Howard Friedman and Leslie Martin in the Eight-Decade Study of 1,500 men and women followed into their eighties and nineties: *conscientiousness*. As Friedman and Martin describe, conscientious people "find their way to happier marriages, better friendships, and healthier work situations."

Despite Muriel's long-standing resilience based on both her in-the-moment and lifelong wisdom, her life was still hanging in the balance. Sometimes stresses or trauma can be too much even for our wisest instincts when we edge toward points of no return. The linear pattern of an age point can begin to come undone, with each component turned on its head, going in reverse or sometimes leapfrogging one another. A resolution fails and we fall back into a suspension of belief and emotion. We reckon with a seemingly insurmountable challenge and then another traumatic event occurs, leaving us spinning, failing, and falling into the collapsing abyss of an age point. Some other strength is needed to push or pull us up and beyond what seems to be the event horizon of a black hole. We need a rationale for survival that trumps the particularities of our wisdom and that points us toward the future. We need a sense of *purpose*.

The Power of Purpose

In being resilient, we discover ways to exercise and prove the existence and powers of our abilities, values, and self-worth to ourself and others. This success in the face of adversity is the ultimate act of dignity. It enlivens and rejuvenates us, and is the best action that we can take against our certain mortality. In being resilient we exercise our purpose in life—to not only survive but to *do* something positive and to *gain* something for ourself and the worlds in which we reside. These actions give us hope for what we can do again in the future. We may have begun life with a keen sense of hope and then pursued various purposes as we aged, but in later life we actually prove to ourselves the relevance of this purpose. And for some aging individuals facing an extreme crisis, it's literally a moment to put up their strengths or face a tragic collapse.

The word *purpose* has a static meaning, as an "aim" or "intention," and an active meaning, "to put forth," "to intend," and "to propose." The word immediately conjures up the future as it shows us a direction in which to travel and an existing horizon to pursue. It puts forth a reason or rationale for our lives, giving us meaning so that we are both satisfied and preoccupied with static reasons for *being* and by dynamic tasks to be *doing*. Having a sense of purpose can grow with age given all the time and life experiences we have and the knowledge we accrue, and it can also give us a reason for aging—a fundamental "why" for aging and surviving.

The groundbreaking work of psychologist Dr. Carol Ryff highlights the importance of purpose. She is best known for her development of a model of well-being with six core elements, of which purpose is one of the most important and influential. Carol's work and that of others in the Midlife in the United States (MIDUS) study has shown that having a sense of purpose has a direct positive impact on health and longevity, in part by reducing the incidence of cardiovascular events such as heart attacks and strokes.

In seeking to understand the role of purpose in aging lives, I sought out Carol and asked her where her own drive and inspiration came from. Her background would not have foretold her later passions. She grew up in Wheatland, a small town of about twenty-three hundred people, located 70 miles north of Cheyenne in the flat and sparsely populated High Plains of Wyoming. The people in her community were largely immigrants who survived on ranching and farming, and they struggled, in her words, to make life go well. Carol was the first person in the history of her family to pursue higher education, and it wasn't until well into her adulthood that she discovered another intellectual kindred spirit among them. As it turned out, her grandmother Meta, or "Grammy," had been a closet lover of poetry who used to check out books by the great American poets from the local library. Grammy loved such poets as Walt Whitman, Edna St. Vincent Millay, and the American transcendentalist Ralph Waldo Emerson—a secret in plain sight as she gave the middle name "Ralph" to Carol's uncle and "Waldo" to her father. After her passing, Carol discovered Grammy's small notebooks, into which she had copied poems from many of these bards.

Even without knowing of Grammy's intellectual yearnings, Carol always saw her as a positive female role model who found time to exercise her great talents for playing the piano, knitting, and crocheting while raising multiple children during the Great Depression out in the "wilderness" of Wyoming. Carol regrets not knowing the intellectual voice of her grandmother, but she now sees herself as a co-traveler for its expression, musing that "there was so much inside of her that she didn't talk about. . . . Maybe some of that now speaks through me." Seeing both the struggles and the beauty in the lives of those around her inspired a certain questioning in Carol as to what the good life is all about. What is the best that we can be, Carol asked—vital and contributing, vibrant and resilient—even in the midst of life's changes and challenges? It's the same question of "why" I pose here in various permutations in my attempt to tap into the basic driving forces and reasons for finding value and meaning in our aging self. Her grandmother quietly sought answers from the great poets—whereas Carol peered into psychology and philosophy. Like myself, she was deeply inspired by the thinking of Erik Erikson, Carl Rogers, Abraham Maslow, Victor Frankl, and others who were all trying to describe positive functioning above and beyond merely being happy. It was clear to her that the integration of these perspectives foretold a pathway to leading a life of meaning and purpose.

The true bolt of lightning, however, occurred when she sat down to read the *Nicomachean Ethics* by Aristotle. She was blown away by how this Greek philosopher from over two thousand years ago was struggling with the same big questions in life that she and countless others have faced; namely, how should one live? This was the same practical question she saw enacted in the lives of the people she grew up with in the prairie and scrub of Wyoming, and later in the intellectual pursuits she encountered in the halls of academia. Aristotle defined the highest of all human activity as experiencing the soul in harmony with the practical virtues of daily life—what he referred to as *eudaimonia*. The term is sometimes translated as "well-being" or "happiness," but its meaning is much richer. For Carol, it refers to a central task in life to come to know our uniqueness as human beings and then strive to work with those capacities and talents to make the most of them. The role of "purpose" in life flows from this concept, as it gives us a way of moving forward that is *mindful* and *virtuous*—meaning that we are aware and in control of it while also concerned about doing good.

As Carol pursued these studies, the role of purpose in life emerged as a core factor in her model of well-being. Looking at aging, in particular, she initially saw a potential roadblock. Some studies have revealed that on average the degree of purpose and personal growth may decline with age—if one looks only at the overall profiles by age. Carol takes a broader view, however, since such scores speak to what is probable and not to what is possible. The MIDUS study has revealed an enormous variation among aging individuals, and has highlighted the fact that those with higher levels of purpose have higher levels of continued personal growth. Moreover, these individuals with high purpose have less cognitive impairment, better physiologic responses to stress, and fewer heart attacks and strokes, and they live longer. This phenomenon holds across cultures; for example, as seen in aging Japanese individuals who have high levels of *ikigai*, or a "reason for living." In short, *purpose is protective.*

Carol is still relatively young at sixty-six years of age, but she is increasingly seeing the power of aging in terms of bringing us a "greater appreciation for the beauty of life" and an "enhanced capacity to find meaning in everything." Having a sense of purpose is both a product of aging and its greatest tool. Without even knowing it, we are healthier because of it. When we hit the bumps and bangs of an age point, we wield it to guide us through to a resolution. In this context, purpose has two faces: one that looks backward into our past and prompts us to accept both the good and the bad—because the other face is simultaneously looking forward and teaching us that our direction, goals, and meaning stem from this past and give us a reason for living. Carol emphasizes that even in the ninth stage, when we are restricted by physical decline and losses, we still have the capacity to appreciate and approach each day with some direction. "It's all about how you frame what you have," she teaches, that even when we seem to have so very little, we have so much.

❦

As Muriel's last days approached, Ellyn called me and pleaded for some suggestions on how to salvage her mom. Hospice care seemed to be the logical approach, but I decided to give one more boost of advice. My message was simple: tell her doctors to cut back on the pain meds and consult with the hospital's psychiatrist to find a way to best treat her delirium. If they could get her through the pancreatitis and mental fog, she had a chance to come to our center and try against all odds to change the course of her situation. Both her daughter and I mustered up a small measure of hope for Muriel, since she had neither the mind nor matter to hope for herself. We knew, however, that Muriel had the potential to survive. And why was that?

Go back and think about how the elements of resilience—both our strengths and vulnerabilities—come together to divine an outcome. Now, turn the equation on its head and ask again the question: Why survive? I have seen and learned from all the people aging around me that we survive simply by doing. We put one foot in front of the other, sometimes based on our own inner compass and other times with a trusted guide. We bend but we don't break. In the process, we see our answer: aging can bring an emerging direction and energy whose sum is greater than its parts. This becomes our purpose in life—an active drive forward in which we seek new knowledge or understandings, connections with others, renewals of the goals and values from our lives, a legacy for the future, and the final and glorious opportunity to create something new and finally "say what we want to say"—to paraphrase the eloquent words of the French artist Henri Matisse in his final years of bursting creativity. Too often we see a mirage of aging as a problem here, bringing all sorts of maladies and tragedies on the shimmering horizon. In reality, aging can be the solution to both the momentary and long-standing stresses of our lives, bringing an ever-expanding reserve of wisdom and a dynamic sense of purpose. It is no surprise, then, that survey after study after survey finds that aging brings less stress and greater well-being to the vast majority of us in our later years. Aging itself gives us the rationale, the tools, the will, and the motivation to keep growing and developing.

So, what happened with Muriel? She survived the pain and the pancreatitis, emerged from a delirium, and made it to our center. She gave up on her previous pain doctor and put herself in the hands of our rehabilitation program, partly on her own accord but also carried by her family. Our pain specialist, Dr. Corbett, reviewed her lengthy and complicated medical history and distilled it down to an elegant plan. She couldn't live without some pain medication, so he devised a regimen that provided enough relief throughout the day while allowing her to be fully awake and functional. This was not palliative care, in his mind, but simply a bridge to a better future. After a few trials and errors, I finally found both an antidepressant and a sleeping pill that would keep Muriel's mood in check while guaranteeing sufficient restorative sleep. These medications did not constitute her main treatment, however, but were necessary and realistic to keep her afloat. The main treatment involved a team of therapists who surrounded Muriel and got her moving, walking and talking every day of the week. It was all about *her*—for once in her life.

As our treatment program unfolded, Muriel's daughter, Ellyn, decided that her mom was too fragile to return to her apartment, and moved her into her multigenerational household to keep a closer eye on her and become *her* caregiver. Muriel was surrounded on a daily basis by her daughter and son-in-law, and was only ten minutes away from her son and several grandchildren who are always swarming the house. I got a text from Ellyn one day with a photo showing Muriel sitting at the kitchen table and leaning forward toward her eight-month-old great-granddaughter, who was reaching out and giggling as she touched Muriel's nose. Both smiling faces—separated by eighty years in time—radiated common joy.

And then, an unexpected but near miraculous event occurred that bolstered Muriel's course even more. Ellyn decided on the spur of the moment to rescue a dog that was otherwise heading for a certain demise. She quickly raced to the kennel, scooped up the young Goldendoodle, and brought it home without even looking at its papers. When she finally had time to open the dog's information, her jaw dropped. Its given name was "Buddy" and it had the exact same birthday as Muriel's beloved husband, Buddy. Muriel took this as a sign from beyond, and the dog became an instant companion. It has so far shredded her checkbook and chewed up many of Muriel's papers—but no matter. She walks him every day (or he walks her) and this supposedly decrepit and dying woman will sometimes be out walking for over an hour with the dog. Muriel the caregiver has risen again.

I saw Muriel the other day, walking down the hallway of our center, leaning on her walker and with the physical therapist next to her, beaming and laughing with me as I beheld a sight I could hardly imagine a few months prior. The lesson about aging that I have learned from countless individuals was evident in this image of Muriel, and also in the course of her life prior and going forward. I've seen why people age, and I've learned how they survive—but that is not often enough. Aging also brings us new possibilities and opportunities to go above and beyond what came before—to renew and reinvent ourselves in creative ways that we might not have imagined before. It's not just about aging and surviving. It's also a time to thrive.

PART III

Why Thrive?

Aging and creativity present an unparalleled opportunity for us as individuals, to grow as we grow older, in ways that in younger years we could not even have dreamed.

—GENE COHEN, *The Creative Age*

Chapter 5

Safety in the Stagnant Quo

THE IMAGES THAT Bodi sent me are from the heyday of his career as a photographer—all selfie-like poses with his famous clientele from an era before selfies were an actual thing. In one photo, he stands arms crossed with a smug grin next to a young Geraldo Rivera, while in another he radiates awe posing next to Coretta Scott King. One of the most impressive photos looks most like an actual selfie, as Bodi appears to be straining to tilt his head into the scene next to the imposing, square-jawed figure of Ted Kennedy, whose serious expression, capped by a royal wave of hair, seems to be staring off the face of a coin. These photos are all from the early to mid-1980s, when Bodi was the king of advertising photography, running a successful studio in midtown Manhattan and managing one of the most recognized ad campaigns of the era.

When Bodi first came to see me a few years ago, however, he was no longer a king. Instead, he reported a long-standing history of depression that was flaring up again after a relatively long dormancy. He had just turned sixty-five, and although this is a common retirement point for many individuals, he felt as if his life had been in the doldrums for many years and now seemed to be stalling even more. His demeanor was always friendly and pleasant, but he wore a sadness on his face and expressed a feeling of boredom and sometimes outright failure. Bodi's life had peaked in his midforties, with incredible personal success in his work that brought in nearly a million dollars in earnings in 1984. The major New York advertising firms wanted Bodi, needed Bodi, and sought out Bodi for their print and TV ad campaigns for products such as M&M cookies, Bic shavers, and his pièce de résistance—IBM's ubiquitous 1980s ads for their new personal computers (PCs) featuring a Charlie Chaplin avatar in tux, top hat, and floppy shoes trying to show how even the lovable Little Tramp could "move with modern times" and bring the power of the PC into each home. Bodi was young, vibrant, and successful—depicted best in the photo he sent me, in which his grinning, confident, and joyful self stands arm in arm with none other than the 1980s prophet of successful aging—comedian George Burns.

So, what happened with Bodi between his peak in 1984 and his rut when he found his way to my office? What factors led to such a dramatic tumble in income and stature, marked depression, and finally a quiet and humble life in South Florida—so far away, it seemed, from the bustle of his former studio throne in Manhattan? When I asked Bodi this very question, he described to me how he failed in his struggle to reinvent himself as the world of advertising photography changed around him. He came to believe that staying on top required something he couldn't get, explaining that "I would have needed a new brain." Like the dawn of a new fashion or music style that washes out the old and sweeps in the new, advertising styles changed and Bodi was no longer the "in" person. He tried over and over, but could not replicate his previous success. In response, he slowly but steadily withdrew into what I call the "stagnant quo" of aging—a life that appears quiet and safe but lacking the creative pursuits or relationships that once brought so much purpose and meaning.

Bodi was relatively young when his world shifted so dramatically, but his experiences are common for many aging individuals who retire, take on new roles, or reach a point where their normally busy and fulfilling life begins to change and they lose their previous pathways and purposes. Sometimes, this change is by choice; other times, it is forced by life circumstances. Either way, it's a disorienting and seminal age point that often comes to define the rest of one's life. Trying to move forward and either renew a previous strength or success or reinvent oneself into something different is often difficult, frightening, and seemingly impossible, and might prompt someone to simply give up. The resulting stagnant quo is safe, reassuring, and sustaining—but also constricting. At best, it brings a relatively quiet life as long as there are no significant stresses or other circumstances that challenge its limits. At its worst, it is represented by rigid and reactionary approaches to aging that can lead to estrangement or outright conflict with others. Examples include aging individuals who cannot move on to new relationships after major losses, who cannot embrace different ways to think or create, or who refuse to try new technology because it seems too complicated or even unnecessary. It's John Henry against the steam drill.

The stagnant quo also drives what some have labeled a "youthist" philosophy among individuals who venerate looking and acting young, as if that is the greater good. Aging people who ignore or deny the changes that come with age and try to maintain or recapture the attributes of their younger self, however, often run into serious roadblocks. In desperation, they may act like aging despots who refuse to yield the grip of power or prestige, and end up driving future generations to ruin. They risk becoming the kind of bickering, backbiting, entitled, and eternally offended people who we see on reality television every day. Ageist attitudes are often reinforced by encounters with such older individuals who refuse to accept change and are stereotyped as "stuck in their ways."

Nonetheless, there is compelling logic to keeping things stable and unchanged as we age. Why not circle the wagons and resist changes that may be painful and destructive? If we've done things a certain way and it's worked well, why change? Even if we've embraced aging and optimized surviving, what else does aging bring? These questions can be condensed into the third and final important question that we face as we age: Why thrive?

Geropause

For middle-aged women, the experience of menopause is a major transition in life. As estrogen production slackens and then ceases, a woman's body feels and shows numerous changes, and her mind must cope with the fact that she is no longer fertile. Men undergoing andropause face mildly comparable changes in their body as testosterone levels slowly decline, with losses in muscle mass, libido, and strength. With both phenomena, aging has come knocking on the door as physical attributes that are fundamental parts of our identity begin to change. In an analogous fashion, the sort of challenging and symbolic stagnant quo–causing age points that Bodi and other aging individuals face can sometimes impose a halt or deviation from previous personal development. This stalled development does not involve the same hormonal or physiological changes as with menopause or andropause, but can have an equal if not more profound symbolic and life-altering impact. This age-associated phenomenon is common but has no specific word to describe it, and so in lieu of the inelegant term *stagnant quo*, I will instead suggest "geropause" as an appropriate label.

A *geropause* refers to a downward shift or even a moratorium on pursuing and developing new interests, skills, relationships, roles, or life circumstances. For many aging individuals, a gero-pause is synonymous with retirement from active creative activi-ties. For an artist, craftsman, or writer, it is a block from previous artistry; literally, the cessation of creative works. Geropause in-volves the loss of one's purpose without anything to replace it. It is not the end of aging per se, but the end of aging that is *dynamic*, meaning that it is a force for change, and the end of aging that is *creative*, meaning that it is generating and innovating new things. In essence, a geropause is the beginning of our stereotypical con-ception of "old age."

The age point that triggers a geropause may occur at the brink of the adult aging process, as with Bodi, or much later in the pro-cess, as with a woman I'll call Suzanne. Suzanne's life up until the age of seventy-two had been what she described as a "good hec-tic," working as a fund-raiser for several charities, traveling with her husband, and spending time with her grandchildren. After her beloved father died, she decided it was time to retire from work and devote more time to her mother. Unfortunately, she discov-ered that her husband was having an affair, and during an attempt to reconcile with him it became apparent that there had been too many secrets and lies for her to trust him again. In grief, she moved away to live near her daughter, buoyed in part by memories of her wonderful younger years as a doting mother. This attempt to renew her role as a mother was ill-fated from the get-go, however, since her son-in-law kept her at arm's length.

Within ten months of her move, Suzanne found herself running out of funds and feeling increasingly depressed. She returned to her home state and temporarily moved in with her elderly mother, only to find herself in perpetual conflict with her brother. She was at a major crossroads in her life, but felt paralyzed over what to do. The crown of wisdom that she had gained with age—all the self-knowledge, caring instincts, and insights into her family dynamics—was now not a strength but a lodestone around her neck, making her feel even more depressed, inadequate, and bereft of support. She had grown up with a lifelong model of being a woman who got married, had kids, and ran a family—but this perceived "normal" situation was at odds with her current life circumstances. The strong men in her life had all abandoned her, and she grieved each loss—by death, by affair, by rejection—every day. She fretted about losing her ninety-year-old mother. She was swallowed in a geropause—stuck in time and place, wanting to feel better, but not certain who, what, or where would make the difference.

The circumstances of both Bodi and Suzanne illustrate different forms of a geropause depending on how it is triggered and perpetuated.

Active: An *active* geropause occurs when someone makes a conscious decision to retire from work or to stop an endeavor, relationship, or pursuit, with the expected but not fully realized consequences that a major cessation of previous activity and purpose will occur. Examples include retiring from a job without a clear plan B, ending a marriage without any plans for seeking other relationships, or quitting a church or club without any new connections in sight.

Passive: A *passive* geropause occurs when someone loses motivation, purpose, opportunities, resources, skills, or some other ability that was key to sustaining his or her activity. Examples include losing interest in the beliefs of one's religion, no longer having sufficient eyesight or coordination to keep driving, or running out of money to keep paying for a club membership or regular vacations.

Inhibited: An *inhibited* geropause results from the rapid imposition of fears, lack of confidence, or some conflict that blocks previous activities. Examples include becoming afraid to drive on highways and so ceasing to go to an adult education program, feeling one can't play bridge as well as before and so no longer attending regular tournaments, or dropping out of an organization after having a fight with members of the board.

In each type of geropause, a person has refused or is unable to change or confront a barrier, leading him or her to withdraw into a more limited and protective lifestyle. The narrow and constricted circumstances of a geropause can be a recipe for unhappiness, boredom, or turmoil, however, if the person becomes dissatisfied with his or her situation or has new stresses or demands imposed by its unintended circumstances. For example, Suzanne believed that moving in with her mother would be simple and economical, allowing her to relax with a loving relative and build up some cash reserves. After a few months, however, she learned that her family was not willing to help with any care issues or finances, and so the burden fell squarely on Suzanne and quickly became overwhelming and demoralizing.

Both Bodi and Suzanne initially tried but failed to get out of their geropause, and this realization led to feelings of frustration and eventually depression. In their cases, as with all geropauses, there are three fundamental factors that drive such failures—*nostalgia*, *old brain*, and *friction*.

Nostalgia: The term *nostalgia* refers to an emotional yearning for a place, time, or circumstances from one's past that one perceives to have brought great personal satisfaction, happiness, and meaning. Nostalgia is an influential psychological phenomenon whose power can be found in its very origins in the Greek terms *nóstos*, which means "homecoming," and *álgos*, which means "ache" or "pain." The term was originally used to describe the homesickness in ancient soldiers. Research has shown that a nostalgic point of view can counteract loneliness, help us cope with stress, improve our mood, enhance meaning, and increase our perceptions of being supported, all by transporting our mind to places of comfort and connection. The construction of a nostalgic point of view, as with all memories of the past, does not necessarily have to jibe with what actually existed or occurred, but is largely a motivated, contrived set of memories that can change over time. Although we imagine memories of the past to be like permanent chiseled inscriptions in our brain, they are actually quite malleable, especially with repeated recollection. Thus, we can conjure up a nostalgic point of view as needed, sculpt it to the circumstances, and feel better about our situation.

In a geropause, however, nostalgia brings all the positive feelings and soothing but also serves as a trap by fixating a person in the past and casting a pall on the present and future as inadequate and even dangerous. The person wants to preserve, experience, and develop a previous world that no longer exists, and which can only exist by pushing aside or denying current reality. C. S. Lewis captured the risk of this pursuit, stating, "These things—the beauty, the memory of our own past—are good images of what we really desire; but if they are mistaken for the thing itself they turn into dumb idols, breaking the hearts of their worshippers. For they are not the thing itself." Cultures that attempt to preserve specific customs from the past have to repeat them endlessly and constantly identify and weed out intrusive elements, which requires a tremendous amount of energy and admonitions on a community level. On a personal level during a geropause, this is tough to do without alienating friends and family.

Consider the case of my former patient Myra who came to me not by choice but on the urging of her daughter. She was seventy-six years old and spent her winters in Miami visiting her daughter while her husband remained in New York. When we met, she denied having any new or different problems other than her long-standing grief over the loss of her eldest son from suicide some twenty years prior. For over an hour she described to me his life in detail, including his success as a stockbroker, his two beautiful children, and his broken marriage, which led to a depression and then death. The details she provided of the days leading up to that last event, and the poisoned relationship with her daughter-in-law, sounded as if they happened a week ago. In her mind, I realized, the events were still quite raw even after two decades. She lived her life based on this loss, and attempted to impose her grief and what she imagined to be her son's wishes and values on his two children, who were now adults themselves. Her relationship with her husband was frozen in time and had never grown beyond her grief, and so she spent little time with him. Her daughter was growing increasingly concerned because her mother refused to do anything other than talk about her dead son and try to spend time with his children. It was an obsession that had not yielded to several attempts at psychotherapy over the years. The daughter felt neglected and was worried that her brother's two children were becoming sick of their grandmother's intrusive style, especially as they were about to begin their own families.

Myra's nostalgia for her life when her son was still alive was soothing her mourning, even after so many years, but was crippling and stunting every other relationship and pursuit in her life. She did reasonably well when she could step in as a second mother to his children, but this would eventually come to an end. Her connection to her son and the world in which he was alive was beginning to fray, but she remained stuck. Somehow, she needed to find a way beyond her grief—but she viewed such a change as synonymous with having to give up and finally lose her son. To Myra, such a thought was simply unthinkable.

Old brain: Bodi's comment about needing a "new brain" was telling. Our brain is socialized in a given time, place, and culture and becomes wired in certain ways as a result. The "greatest generation," as they are called, have common views on service to country and the role of patriotism that tend to be different from those of individuals who grew up during the Vietnam War era. They grew up on big band music whereas their children grew up with rock and roll; they grew up with traditional roles of men and women, whereas their children led the women's liberation movement and the sexual revolution. These cohort effects lay down general ways of thinking and feeling about life that can be difficult to break. Bodi became successful as a photographer by breaking from previous styles and introducing a new approach; but then younger photographers came in with a "new brain" that pushed him and others aside. If such "old brains" can't think like newer brains, they must instead be willing to do different things, perhaps even by giving up previous vocations. Bodi still wanted to be an advertising photographer but couldn't imitate new styles, and so he failed at the same profession. He was able to find some success as an art dealer, but never with the same personal or financial success as he had before. He was not able to adjust both his profession and expectations, and this perpetuated his geropause.

Friction: Sometimes change brings too much psychological or interpersonal emotion, conflict, or overall friction to bear, and a person withdraws so as to lessen the pain. In these circumstances, there is often a lack of sufficient will, grit, and self-confidence. Psychologist Albert Bandura referred to this attribute as "self-efficacy," or the belief in one's ability to complete a task or meet a goal. As we age, we often retain knowledge of our abilities and strengths, but sometimes lose confidence in our ability to exercise them. This loss of self-efficacy prompts fears of failure and loss of dignity, which in turn fuels the paralysis of a geropause. Many individuals who once thrived in a marriage or other relationships often give up after being divorced or widowed, not feeling able or confident enough to be able to engage in a mutual caring, affectionate, and even sexual relationship in later life. They imagine the friction of misunderstandings, rejections and the potential burden of romantic or sexual needs and decide that it's simply not worth it; indeed, that it is easier and better to be alone. This is not to imply that every aged person who is single is in a geropause, but to point out that sometimes the decision to be alone is guided less by personal preference and more by fear.

Several core fears of a geropause are driven by a combination of these factors. For example, if you ask aging people how to troubleshoot issues with a personal computer or smartphones, they often point to an adult child or grandchild as their information technology specialist. Never before in history have older generations been so dependent on younger generations for technological guidance. In ancient tribes, the adults and elders taught the main customs— how to hunt, skin animals, sew, and prepare meals. Throughout all subsequent history, the transfer of knowledge from old to young didn't reverse until the 1980s, when newer, smaller, and faster pieces of technology began emerging on a regular basis, many linked to the use of music or games that are of primary interest to adolescents and young adults.

As I observe aging individuals struggle with newer technology (myself included), I often hear a *nostalgia* for simpler times when one's world was shaped by the morning newspaper, the radio, and phone calls on a landline. I encounter *old brains* that are confused by the array of tasks that a smartphone can accomplish, having grown up in an analog era when machines were capable of fewer things that often had to be dialed in or set up ahead of time. I also see the confusion, frustration, and overall *friction* of aging people's trying to move between photos, texts, and apps on a smartphone. In our fast-paced digital world, there are an increasing number of individuals in their eighties and nineties who are in a functional geropause because they refuse to even consider using computers, smartphones, and the Internet to help communicate with others and manage their life.

On the whole, these individuals are not modern-day Luddites or technophobes. They do not actively reject new technology or its cultural manifestations, such as social media, because they see it as a threat to their worldview. According to Dr. Sarah Czaja, a psychologist and human factors engineer and the director of the Center on Aging at the University of Miami Miller School of Medicine, they may reject it or not engage with it because they do not perceive its potential value or they do not have adequate access or support for setting up and maintaining it. Czaja has learned that aging individuals often have a deeper appreciation for the inherent value of newer technology when they immerse themselves in it and lend their voice to its design and implementation. The depth of their interest contrasts with that of younger people who are enamored by the latest gadget because it is, well, the latest gadget. Technological geropauses will occur, however, when aging individuals lack the self-efficacy to engage with newer technologies or when they are excluded from the development process by ageist attitudes harbored by younger engineers and designers.

Is There a Way Out?

Bodi brought his geropause to my doorstep, but he also showed me a way out. It was a long journey, with its roots deep in his personal history. He was born at the end of World War II in Brussels to a Belgian Walloon mother and a Ukrainian expatriate father who had fled the Russian revolution in the early 1920s. His father was an intellectual who preferred reading papers and books to actually working and was not well liked by his mother's family, to whom he was frequently in debt. His mother was a skilled dressmaker who did her best to keep food on the table during a period of postwar rationing. Bodi remembers his first twelve years growing up in Belgium as full of deprivation, with meager food, little money, and few toys or any other possessions. In 1958, Bodi and his parents and two sisters immigrated to the United States to escape poverty, debt, and the general dislike of his father's mother's family. His first memory of arriving on the docks in New York City was finding an errant five-dollar bill and thinking that America was literally paved with money.

His happy discovery was somewhat of a seminal event for Bodi, as he realized that any success in life would have to come through his own eyes and hands. His father was a distant figure who rarely provided for the family or expressed love. His mother was more interactive but not an especially affectionate woman. Nonetheless, she worked hard as a seamstress for the fashion industry, and was the family's main provider. Bodi recalls her expert ability to copy dress designs from the Paris fashion shows, which made her a highly skilled asset for any house of haute couture.

In high school, Bodi first began working with cameras, and it became his passion. Photography came naturally to him, and he loved to study its techniques and immerse himself in the art and process of developing, going so far as to set up his own basement darkroom. His exceptional talent caught the attention of his art teacher, who mentored and inspired him to consider photography as a profession. On the basis of his impressive portfolio of photographs, Bodi was accepted to the prestigious Art Center College of Design in Pasadena, what he likened to the "Harvard" of photography. Part of his ticket to acceptance was an award-winning photo he took of a statue of Christopher Columbus in Central Park, with the sun bursting from behind its bronze head.

The art college was an incredible opportunity for Bodi but extremely intense, requiring night after night working on excessively detailed projects, many of which didn't involve the sort of photography that interested him the most. Before too long he ran out of both money and energy, and returned to Manhattan to start pursuing his career in photography. Bodi began working as an assistant to a photographer and then went out on his own as a freelancer. In those years before digital cameras and design software gave everyone access to great technology, Bodi described good photographers as kings, and he was determined to earn his own crown. As he gained experience and made more connections, he slowly but steadily built up his skills and reputation, until he finally got his own Manhattan studio in the mid-1970s.

He focused on advertising work, doing photo illustrations of brands of beauty treatments, coffee, liquor, and many other products. His own style began to replace the generation before him, as he began creating elaborately staged scenes full of color and movement that broke from the staid, Norman Rockwell–like scenes that were now becoming passé. He knew the tricks to getting the lighting just right to bring out the desired colors, and how to coax and capture the exact facial expressions that the art directors imagined. A bevy of celebrities and politicians flowed through his studio— Wilt Chamberlain, Henry Kissinger, and James Earl Jones, among many others. He created both whimsical scenes and dramatic portraits, and traveled the country to conduct elaborate photo shoots. And then in 1982 he signed a huge five-year contract with IBM to create dozens of ads featuring a Charlie Chaplin character interacting with the company's new personal computer. It was an unparalleled success—so much so that when I first met Bodi and learned about his work, I vividly remembered seeing those ads back in high school and college when I was enamored by the idea of having my own computer. Partly influenced by Bodi's artistic vision, IBM became the cool computer before Apple's stylistic takeover.

Bodi soared for about five years before the slow crash began. After a peak in 1984, earnings lessened each year as fewer jobs came his way. He could see styles begin to change. Art directors at the major advertising firms began looking for looser, less staged photos. These changes forced him to reckon with his field: "Advertising is a form of visual lies," he related to me, "and after a while people associate the style with the lie and it stops working unless, of course, the style is changed. But that's how I was able to get in because the old guard's work was going out of style. I displaced a lot of people when I came into it." Now it was Bodi's turn to be replaced. Advertising was a harsh field that consumed one generation and spit out the bones when it hungered for something new. Bodi was now the bones.

At first, Bodi became depressed and nearly suicidal, since his work was always the essence of his self-esteem. He studied the new photographic styles and tried to re-create them, making elaborate storybooks to take around to advertising firms. The art directors were impressed, but they didn't hire him. They cared more about newer styles than experience. He knew what had to be done to capture their interest, but didn't have the requisite abilities of the younger and fresher artistic brains they were seeking. After many failed attempts to resurrect his studio, Bodi closed shop and set out for something new. He spent several years running art galleries and then working for an art publisher. He had modest success with each endeavor but they ended quickly and didn't bring the degree of professional success, personal satisfaction, or income that he had previously enjoyed. Bodi was divorced and had a girlfriend for a while but never remarried. He had few funds to travel to New York to visit his daughter and grandchildren on any sort of regular basis.

When Bodi first came to see me, he was feeling restless and barely making ends meet. His financial pressures appeared, more than anything, to trigger nostalgic thoughts for his glory days in Manhattan, when he was enlivened and enriched by his own creativity and feted by the advertising gods of the day. Still, he did not appear to make much progress, and the quiescent embers of his geropause did not reveal themselves. After several years, however, they began to spark.

He mentioned to me that he was working on something new. "What was that?" I inquired—"Can you show me?" Acceding to my request, Bodi came into my office carrying an oversize laptop computer and holding a long, rolled-up canvas under his arm. He looked the part of a hip Miami artist, with a tousled mop of slightly grayed copper brown hair; round red-framed spectacles; and wearing a bright yellow guayabera, white linen pants, and his signature blue suede shoes. He was more relaxed than I had seen him before, and had a look of excitement on his face as he set up the computer on my desk. "I decided that I want to get back into the art world," he told me. "Why now?" I inquired. "I started thinking that I am ending," he told me. "Even if I live another twenty years, I am still at the end section of life. And what am I leaving behind? Who will remember me? I just can't leave like that. I have a need to leave something behind." Bodi's existential question here was not "Why age?" or "Why survive?" but a clarion call to himself: "Why thrive?" And his answer—*to create something new as his legacy*.

He then showed me the artistic creations that were consuming his time and firing dreams of a showing in a gallery one day soon. He had assembled dozens of his photographs from over the years— many of which he had taken as a young man in the early 1970s— and had begun juxtaposing them in pairs onto a single frame. In one shot, for example, a black-and-white photo on the left showed a line of hippos walking into a pool at the Bronx Zoo, while the colorful shot on the right showed a line of women emerging from church in their Sunday finest. In another, a black-and-white photo of a pudgy, smiling baby held up close to the camera was placed next to a color photo of the empty lot of a gas station.

Bodi had begun creating these photographic combinations in a seemingly random manner as a proof, he contends, that you don't need an inherent relationship between two photos. But he wasn't satisfied with images alone, and began taking small hand-written snippets from old letters from a previous girlfriend and superimposing them on the collages. As I began reading the added words, it was difficult for me as a psychiatrist with a particularly psychodynamic bent not to begin reading some meaning into Bodi's "random" combinations. "It's autobiographical," he admitted, "but like an unfinished painting. Adding the words makes a difference." For example, the words added to the baby–gas station collage read: "I'm scared but it's my chance to do something on my own." I read those words and one eye sees a smiling baby ready to greet the world and the other sees an empty gas station, its pumps primed to fuel a run. There is fear but also opportunity in this artwork—like the artist in Bodi who is emerging from a long hibernation to begin creating anew. Flashing the same face of joy seen in the photo with George Burns, Bodi unfurled the large canvas emblazoned with one of his photographic creations. It was ready for the gallery wall.

As Bodi began to talk about his art, I could see the end of his geropause: "In the past, I didn't have the need to do it. Now it feels freer and more positive. It feels great doing it. Even on days that I work all day long on the computer and come out with nothing—it's still positive." As he sorts through the photos from his past, he often feels twinges of sadness when he encounters a particularly nostalgic scene, such as one in which he was picking up his young daughter from school. But now the nostalgia is not just soothing him but also fueling his creativity—and this creativity brings him great meaning.

Bodi has discovered the essential answer to the question that nearly every person faces in life. As we age, the many roles, skills, and pursuits in our life change and we must either change with them and look for new ways of thinking and doing, or withdraw into safe and well-worn pathways of a geropause that can freeze us in time, limit us, and yet pose great risks of shattering ourselves or those around us when circumstances demand more than we are able or willing to give. Why should we even attempt to go beyond these perceived limitations and actually thrive? *We thrive so as to create something new*, which in turn brings great meaning into our lives and those around us.

Chapter 6

Renewal, Reinvention, and Creative Aging

There are no ordinary people. You have never talked to a mere mortal.

—C. S. LEWIS, *The Weight of Glory*

THERE IS A concept in childhood development called the "good enough parent." Developed by British pediatrician and psycho-analyst D. W. Winnicott in the 1950s, this term refers to a mother or father who provides his or her young child with sufficient attention and affection to enable healthy development despite the expected deficiencies and failures of parenting. It's a way of saying that no parent is perfect, but there is a certain threshold at which we do enough to keep things moving along in the right direction. There is a parallel concept in gerontology called "successful aging." First studied and popularized in the late 1990s by John Rowe and Robert Kahn, the term outlines three components to success in later life: avoiding or minimizing the risk of disease and disability, maintaining high mental and physical functioning, and actively engaging in meaningful life activities. It's a way of saying that no aging person is perfect, but he or she can be successful by maintaining a good enough degree of fitness and activity despite the expected decrepitudes and failures of aging.

Although the term has been critiqued and revised in various ways, it captures an essential truth of how many people would like to age—without much disability and with an actively engaged mind and body. This is increasingly possible for healthy aging individuals but not always realistic for others, as it largely ignores the activities and contributions of individuals who have failed the test—who have significant disease and disability, impaired mental and physical functioning, and limited activities—but who are still aging with purpose and meaning. In addition, the model completely leaves out those in the ninth stage. These blind spots are important to consider since they expose a risky perspective on aging that makes success contingent upon a narrow set of values. As a result, the failure to age successfully under the model sets up the belief that aging beyond a certain point is no longer valuable or meaningful; it is more of a burden that can ethically be neglected or even terminated.

A broader perspective can be found in the concept of "positive aging" proposed and developed by psychologist Robert Hill. In his view, the best quality of an aging life is supported by a state of mind that is positive, optimistic, courageous, and able to adapt and cope in flexible ways with life's changes. Positive aging is affected by disease and disability, but not contingent upon avoiding it. It represents the ways in which we actively manage the good and the bad that aging brings us. The SOC model of aging developed by the gerontologists Paul and Margret Baltes describes one way of positive aging. In the face of age-related decline, we engage in a process of *selection* among various pursuits so as to focus on the ones most relevant, accessible, and meaningful; we work on *optimization* of our abilities through extra rehearsal or exercise; and we adjust our activities or performance to allow for *compensation* in the face of certain deficits. The Balteses and others have cited the example of the aging pianist Arthur Rubinstein, who dealt with age-induced declines in his skills by selecting a more limited repertoire, optimizing his performance through extra practice, and compensating by altering his tempo during certain sections to highlight the dynamics of a piece.

Successful and positive aging tell us how we can both survive and change in the face of an aging process defined by decline and loss, but they do not cast aging itself as a source of strength or solutions. They do not tell us much about how we can *thrive*, which means "to grow strong and vigorously" and "to do well" and "prosper." This term comes from the Old Norse word, *thrifask*, which means "to grasp for oneself," implying an active reaching out and bringing something into one's hands. It is a synonym of *flourish*, which indicates energy, growth, and excellence. To thrive as one ages means to actively grow as a person and develop new pathways and pursuits. To thrive is to reach forth and discover, and achieve or create something above and beyond what came before.

A third major perspective on aging captures this notion of thriving, and that is Gene Cohen's model of *creative aging*. As a geriatric psychiatrist, Cohen was schooled in every aspect of both normal and abnormal or pathological aging, but he was always able to see a higher value, purpose, or accomplishment in aging regardless of its apparent state. He saw not only what aging *is*, but what aging *could be*; not what we accomplish *in spite of aging*, but *because of aging*. He entered the field of aging at a time when it was disdained; in fact, upon hearing of his interest, one of his supervisors suggested he go into psychoanalysis *as a patient*. Undaunted, Gene became one of the founding fathers of geriatric psychiatry. There is a story from his past that speaks to his passion, empathy, and vision. As a young resident in psychiatry, he consulted at a senior housing complex with aged individuals with mental health issues, many of whom had been released from long-term psychiatric hospitals during the push for deinstitutionalization in the late 1960s and early 1970s. Prior to beginning this assignment, he harbored many of the negative stereotypes of aging that were common to his era.

What Gene encountered, however, was unexpected and affirming: "Instead of what others warned would be the most depressing of patients, these elderly men and women proved to be among the most alert, attentive, and responsive—a satisfying kind of patient for a doctor who cares." Gene saw the challenges of aging and mental illness, but he also saw potential. He encountered individuals who did better when they were provided with resources and treatment. As he started looking deeper, he saw more than mere survival—he saw growth and development. He saw new abilities and interests emerge. He saw the dynamic and transformative role of creativity in their lives.

In contrast to everything else written about aging to date, Gene's focus on creative aging was monumental. He suggested that creativity could open our potential in later life by challenging and enabling us to think about things in different ways, to see possibility instead of problems. Creativity was essential to artistic expression, but was also a broad force such that "the secret of living with one's entire being is the creative spirit that dwells in each of us." Cohen outlined four fundamental ways in which creativity can benefit aging: it strengthens our morale, improves our physical health, enriches relationships, and establishes our legacy. Fundamentally, he believed that aging itself was the catalyst to enhance creativity: "It can occur at any age and under any circumstances, but the richness of experience that age provides us magnifies the possibilities tremendously."

To illustrate creative aging, Cohen liked to tell stories of influential individuals who found ways to renew their passions and reinvent themselves in later life. These stories, coupled with my own observations and encounters with patients and other aging individuals, spell out several core lessons about aging and thriving that flesh out Cohen's theory and make the point clearly that aging brings strengths. They show us how age can help us to both renew and reinvent ourselves in the face of inescapable changes.

Lesson 1: The Past Can Help Us Renew Ourselves

It was the winter of 1941, and a seventy-one-year-old man was heading into a disastrous old age. Incessant bouts of severe abdominal pain forced a risky surgery that left him languishing in bed and delirious for months on end. He defied initial predictions of death, but was left wheelchair bound and unable to work in his usual manner. German troops overran his beloved France, tearing asunder the multicolored pieces of his world and sending them to destruction or exile. As the war years advanced, recurrent infections, pain, and anorexia ravaged his body. He had no close family: his wife had left him years before and his daughter was later arrested and tortured nearly to death by the Gestapo. Old age seemed a betrayal of everything he held sacred, leaving him physically disabled and decrepit, isolated, and uncertain of his future. A review of his life in those years could easily lead one to cast being "old" as a curse, a dreaded decline, or a tragic gathering in and then a passing on.

Advance the clock now to the autumn of 2014, when the Paris fashion runways were bursting with color. Models adorned with vibrantly hued fabric cutouts pieced into the latest designs of Christian Dior sashayed to thumping techno music and the cheers and calls of the audience. This brash and stylish couture left critics swooning, and was directly inspired, it must be noted, by one withered old man who had been lying half-dead in a hospital bed some seventy-three years earlier. Something remarkable had emerged from the fading old age of the man in question that continues to have profound influence on modern art, fashion, advertising, and culture. It came from the aged life of an individual who had once been written off as half-dead, with his old age imagined as the beginning of the end. In the life of our protagonist, however, who I now reveal as famed French artist Henri Matisse, we shall see how the maligned oldness ended and age became a dominant strength.

So, how did Matisse do it? How did he return from delirium and near death and manage to revolutionize the art world? The nuns who nursed him back to health in the spring of 1941 called Matisse "*le résuscité*"—the man who rose from the dead. His survival was unexpected and his recuperation was long and tortuous. He spent most of his time either bedbound or in a wheelchair and was unable to stand and stretch his body to paint on large canvases as before. The man who emerged, however, was clear-minded and determined to move forward: "It's like being given a second life," Matisse wrote to his son Pierre, "which unfortunately can't be a long one." As he lay in bed during those long months, Matisse might have been inspired by a profound memory from his youth. At the age of twenty, he was similarly confined to bed for many months as he recuperated from an intestinal ailment. Inspired by his roommate and enabled by a gift of brushes, paints, and canvas from his mother, Matisse first began to paint, and it sparked a lifelong passion: "From the moment I held the box of colours in my hand, I knew this was my life," Matisse wrote, describing himself "like an animal that plunges headlong towards what it loves, I dived in" and discovered a "Paradise Found in which I was completely free, alone, at peace."

Even in the midst of debility and pain, the aged Matisse was able to return to his art with several commissioned projects, buoyed by a rich correspondence with friends. He started slowly, drawing on the wall next to his bed and illuminating letters and postcards to friends. These writings, full of "boisterous jokes, gossips and ragging" made him feel connected with others and papered "over the cracks of old age—infirmities, ailments, setbacks, loneliness, despondency, fear." Matisse also developed a genius way to "paint" as never before. His devoted assistant, Lydia Delectorskaya, would bring vividly colored sheets of paper to the great artist and he would glide a pair of scissors through them, cutting out free-flowing, undulating shapes, or "decorations," as he called them, evocative of appendages, flowers, and ferns. He would then direct his assistant to pin them up in various designs on large colored canvases or on the walls. The results were stunning, with their glowing, luminous colors reminiscent of the beautiful and refined fabrics woven by his ancestors in northern France, and their shapes celebrating the freedom of movement and spirit in postwar Europe. Matisse's new style of paper cutouts first appeared in a book called *Jazz* published in 1947, and consisted of a mélange of acrobats, circus performers, and animals all rendered in bold cutouts. Perhaps the most famous image is Matisse's rendering of the mythical Icarus with his bulbous black body and brilliant red rounded heart splayed against a dark blue sky and lit up by several yellow starbursts. The image is equally symbolic of an aging Matisse, perhaps plunging toward earth and dying, or maybe simply reclining peacefully against an illuminated sky, his heart still beating furiously.

There are two magnificent elements to Matisse's resurrection that speak to the power of aging. First, his cutouts were simultaneously an expression of continuity from his entire past body of work, while also a radical new approach to art. Second, there was a spirit of boldness and freedom in his works that made them so compelling compared to anything that had come before. Matisse was clear that the secret force that enabled this departure was aging: "Even if I could have done, when I was young, what I am doing now—I wouldn't have dared." Age brought him courage and enhanced his creativity. His final masterpiece, created shortly before his death in 1952, was a completely designed chapel in Vence, France, dedicated to the nurse turned nun who cared for him after his surgery. The sublime shapes and colors of the stained-glass windows reflect the essential gift of aging that Matisse articulated so well: "I have needed all that time to reach the stage where I can say what I want to say." This is a powerful statement that every aging person should be able to embrace.

We learn from Matisse and many others our first essential lesson of creative aging: the process of renewal can be life-affirming and lifesaving. It involves reaching out to the best from our past to recapitulate parts of it, revise other parts, and redo them—but in a new context. Matisse himself described how his past helped in the creation of the Vence chapel: "It is the whole of me," he wrote, "everything that was best in me as a child." He preserved the essential memories and ideas from his past but recast them into something new. We may fear change and the unknowns of aging, but renewal reassures us and bolsters us with our memories and wisdom, even as it demands that we rework them.

Lesson 2:
The Present Can Help Us Reinvent Ourselves

No old body is as lithe or limber as its younger form. Tendons shorten and stiffen with age, stretching frayed and weakened muscles across thinning bones and arthritic joints. These changes are noticeable and a nuisance to the average elder, but they were devastating to a seventy-four-year-old dancer who could no longer perform to her own standards, not to mention those of her critics. In response, she slunk away from the stage in 1970 after fifty years of success, later stating that "there comes a time when a work has to be retired." But dancing was her identity, and she could neither comprehend nor cope with her life as the retired work. For four years, her health slowly dissolved into a self-induced exile of depression and alcohol, and in desperation she decided to end it all. The suicide of a seemingly washed-up old woman might not prompt a label of tragedy. After all, she was living beyond the point where ethicist Ezekiel Emanuel urges us to consider whether "our consumption is worth our contribution" in life.

Advance the clock now to 1991, twenty-one years after our older protagonist's somber self-reflection gave way to suicidal impulses. Onstage at New York's City Center, a world-famous dance company performed *The Eyes of the Goddess* and other works. The stage was starkly designed, save for a drab cart with a protruding tree about which the critic noted: "Barren, it nonetheless carries the promise of renewal." In the show's final piece, the aged dancer Mikhail Baryshnikov leapt onto the stage and gave a brilliant, career-defining performance. All the remarkable, stunning choreography had been created by the dance company's eponymous founder, who died only months before at the age of ninety-six. Having survived a suicide attempt some twenty-one years earlier, our aged heroine—renowned dancer Martha Graham—had resurrected her career by shifting from dancer to choreographer and from principal to producer so as to engage and enjoy a long and celebrated encore to her career. As with Matisse, we see how something remarkable happened between the death spiral and swan song of old age—a period of rebalancing and blossoming, even amid loss and decline.

As with Matisse, we must ask the question of how Graham managed not only to survive, but to thrive. The survival part came along while she was lying in her hospital bed, having just emerged from a coma. She had reached what seemed to be an inescapable age point that would result in her death, first from dancing and then from life. But then something mysterious and yet predictable occurred—her life force kicked in and the strengths of aging began to speak: "Then one morning, I felt something welling up within me. I knew that I would bloom again. That feeling, an errand into the maze, over and over in my mind, sustained me to go on. It was the only way to escape the constant fear of what might come." Graham thus began with an image of the future—a glimmer of hope for herself and her underlying abilities. To do so, she first reached back to one of her most famous creations, called *Errand into the Maze*, a dance that conjures up the Greek myth of the labyrinth and the fearsome half-man, half-bull Minotaur who ruled its hidden pathways. In the dance, an eerie, syncopated music plays as the female protagonist steps and twists along a rope maze leading to a large wishbone-shaped aperture, where she is confronted by a leaping bull-horned male dancer. With each successive go-around with the Minotaur-like dancer, she grows less fearful and more confident, and eventually conquers him as he falls to the ground and drops the stick held between his arms. The music softens as she has now conquered her fears, and she stands boldly between the appendages of the aperture, caressing its sides and twisting her leg back and forth, in and out, until she steps through, her arms raised in triumph.

Even as she emerged from her deathbed, the choice for Graham was difficult. No longer able to be the dancer or the designer of the dance based on her own innovative movements, she had to step back and create from a new vantage point. She had to reinvent herself as a choreographer who was creating for others and not for herself. She also had to stop drinking alcohol and find new ways to be resilient by coping with dependency and stress. She had to fight against critics and those in her own company who didn't want her back. One can still watch YouTube videos of the young Martha Graham in many of her signature dances as well as the aged, dignified Martha Graham sitting in the choreographer's chair, wearing a deep purple gown and black gloves, with her hair pulled back in a dancer's bun, as she instructs her dance company in the making of *Maple Leaf Rag*, one of her last creations. In her memoir, *Blood Memory*, she speaks to her fortitude and purpose, writing that even in the anticipation of failure and impending death, "It is the now that I must face and want to face." Age speaks forcefully here: "But what is there for me but to go on? That is life for me. My life." And how did she find the ability to reinvent herself? "How does it all begin?" she asked. Her answer conjures the power of aging: "I suppose it never begins. It just continues."

Martha Graham and others teach us a second essential lesson about creative aging. We cannot forget our past, but often must tap into it for strength and inspiration. At the same time, we cannot always continue the same roles, pursuits, or passions when they depend on elements that change with time, such as our physical dexterity and endurance. At those points of change or loss, we must try something new, either as an extension of what we did before or perhaps in a new direction. We must be willing to let go of certain elements of our past and embrace a new identity. This reinvention of who we are and how we associate with others begins slowly but builds momentum with time. In the end, it allows us to escape from petrified and paralyzing elements of our life that inhibit our development.

Creative Aging

In my work and research, I have encountered countless friends, colleagues, and patients who have chosen to reinvent themselves in life—and done so successfully. Consider the actress Julie Newmar, who graciously offered to speak to me about her own aging experiences. She had a brilliant career as an actress and dancer onstage and in such movies as *Seven Brides for Seven Brothers* as well as her noteworthy portrayal of the sultry Catwoman in the *Batman* TV series of the 1960s. In her later years, her career was limited by physical disability from a neurological condition, but she reinvented herself as a writer, blogger, and social media star with over 130,000 followers on Facebook. Although she is known for her beautiful, sexy persona on the screen, anyone who spends a few minutes speaking to the now eighty-four-year-old Newmar realizes the profound strengths that transcend this persona, as an intellect and a savant on many topics and as a loving and creative caregiver for her disabled son.

Psychologist Christopher Hertzog studies cognitive development in adults and talked to me about age-related changes in intellectual and emotional abilities of the brain. During the course of the interview, I discovered that the sixty-four-year-old Dr. Hertzog is both a new parent to a three-year-old son as well as a long-standing parent to two adult children. This aging soccer dad is able to engage the curator's dual roles to give care to his young son and to take care of his own aging self and children. Aging has given him a better appreciation for non-work-related identities that he did not consider when he was a much younger, newly minted father. A common denominator with individuals who have had to reinvent themselves is not only acceptance of age-related changes but the willingness to apply a creative spirit to both past and present elements and abilities in their life. To achieve this, we must consider a much broader definition of creativity.

I Will Just Be the Person That I Am

For perspective on creativity, I turn to a prominent seventy-year-old dancer and choreographer named Liz Lerman who was the founder of a contemporary dance company called the Dance Exchange and a 2002 recipient of a MacArthur "Genius Grant" fellowship.

Lerman's works are characterized by their frequent inclusion of multigenerational dancers and focus on scientific themes. She has even involved nursing home residents in dance productions. Lerman characterizes reinvention as a daily activity based on constant creating, testing, and revising. In fact, this consummate creative choreographer has reinvented herself as an academic on the full-time faculty at Arizona State University. She lives in the dance department and works across disciplines as a professor for all the arts.

In her book *Hiking the Horizontal*, she outlines creativity as requiring a person to make new and unexpected connections with the worlds of others, to embrace and study paradoxical ideas, to get out of his or her own personal perspectives, and to see discomfort as a fuel for further inquiry. Creativity involves redefining and enlarging a situation by bringing in different people and perspectives. Creativity can be difficult, grinding, frustrating, and sometimes fruitless, but the process inches us forward, and brings new ideas and solutions. Ultimately, it gives us a sense that we are realizing our unique purpose in life, which brings a deep, gut-satisfying sense of meaning.

Renewing and reinventing ourselves are forms of creative aging that really bring out our potential and show the strengths of aging. Lerman, for example, learned to drop an old narrative about herself and start over. As an American choreographer, she was always conscious of not performing at one of the major New York dance festivals. She saw this as a detriment to her career and wondered whether there was something wrong with her or her work. At her new academic home, however, no one cares about that. She knows that her colleagues would never see her as diminished because of her self-perceived detriment, and so she no longer cares about it. Such a realization has been liberating and has set her on her way: "I will just be the person that I am," she proclaimed.

Lerman stresses that creativity is not the same as originality, which is rarer. You can set the conditions for creativity and then change it, control it, and teach it. All people are creative from the moment they awake in the morning and throughout the entire day, as they adapt and make decisions. "Creativity comes unbidden," Lerman explains. "You get a spark. An image comes and you are surprised. But if you practice, you can harness and harvest it." Aging itself sparks change, in part, by driving and developing creativity. This belief led Gene Cohen to a radically different scheme of the life cycle compared to Erikson's belief that our main task in late life involves contemplating and ultimately findings acceptance for our achievements to date and the anticipated ending of life. In contrast, Cohen proposed a series of overlapping "human potential phases" as expressions of our ongoing development and growth.

Cohen's model begins with a "midlife reevaluation phase" in our mid- to late thirties through the midsixties, characterized by a newfound motivation to reevaluate our life and make positive changes using what he called "quest energy." Next, we may enter a "liberation phase" in our midsixties to midseventies, which is characterized by a sense of urgency to engage in experimental or innovative activities that were not considered in the past. This phase is often triggered and supported by the freedom of time and openness that comes with retirement. The "summing-up phase" occurs in our late sixties to nineties, and is energized by a desire to contribute to the world and find some significantly larger meaning in life. Finally, there is the "encore phase" in our late seventies to the end of life, which is characterized by activities that restate, reaffirm, and celebrate the major themes in our life. Many individuals have shown me the essence of this model of human potential.

CR

Martin came to me not as a patient but as the husband of a dying woman. His wife, Ella, eighty-seven years old, was suffering from cognitive impairment due to a stroke. Her short-term memory was poor and she could no longer walk. As is common in individuals with significant damage to the lower, subcortical regions of the brain, she was quite apathetic and did not talk much or have any interest or motivation to participate in activities. She preferred to spend most of the day in her bed or reposed in a reclining chair, staring out the window. Her swallowing ability had deteriorated precipitously in the past few months, and she could barely consume even thickened and pureed foods without coughing and choking. When we met, Martin led the discussion with me and his two children on what course should be taken, without Ella present. He had known Ella since junior high; she had always been the one and only love in his life and he defined himself by his role as her partner. This eighty-eight-year-old retired businessman was now Ella's full-time caretaker since her stroke, only giving in and hiring an aide when he could no longer physically lift her to put her in a chair or bring her to the toilet. Despite his distress over her condition, he was clear-headed about her prognosis and did not want to have a feeding tube placed. After he conferred with me and his family, he decided to enroll Ella in hospice care.

Martin's decision was logical, but it seemed unimaginable to me how this husband, partner, and friend of the same woman for over seventy-five years could face such a loss. I worried that his very identity would die along with Ella. In hopes of offering some support, I invited him to come meet with me alone, and we spent a few hours together talking about his life and his future. To anyone who met Martin, he was a relatively nondescript man whose life revolved around his wife. He had several of his own health issues and physical frailties, and by appearance would certainly not light up the board as a vigorous or vibrant person if one met him in a crowd of similarly aged individuals. He was generally quiet and humble and neither his demeanor nor his typical garb of a brown or gray shirt and dark slacks called much attention to him. In fact, his current circumstances might easily lead one to feel pity and dismiss his life as bland, boring, and soon to be tragic.

When I spoke to Martin and really tried to get to know him, however, I was astonished. At first, he was reluctant to talk about himself or his life. I got him to start by describing how he had met Ella. The two of them had lived on the same block, and they fell in love nearly at first sight when the brash, gum-chewing tomboy met the gangly, awkward tinkerer. They started off as admiring friends in junior high, became nearly inseparable by high school, and formulated plans to marry right before Martin donned an army uniform and set off for Europe in the signal corps. As a World War II buff, I pressed Martin on the details of his service, and he was characteristically humble and discreet. "Oh, I worked in the tent of one of the officers," he told me. With a little cajoling, I learned that Martin was a key communications officer in the tent of none other than General George Patton leading up to and during the Battle of the Bulge! In fact, when one learns about all the historical events celebrating Patton, it is important to realize that Martin was usually a few steps away, quietly and efficiently handling many of the critical communications that enabled the war to flow. As wide-eyed as I was about this chapter in Martin's young life, I realized that every single role or responsibility that came afterward, even up to our most recent meeting, was guided by the immense experience and wisdom of this man. As much as we ascribe the great historical events of our age to giants like Patton or other geniuses and charismatic figures, it is actually the diligent and dedicated expertise of men like Martin that makes the clock of progress and history tick forward.

By the end of our discussion, I was nearly exhausted with awe and admiration for Martin. Out of the drab browns and grays of this aged man who once stealthily passed through my clinic, I could now see bursting, vivid colors. For eighty-eight years he had driven, in succession, a war, a marriage, a family, and a business. How could I ever doubt his abilities now? Martin seemed to enjoy our conversation, but after a few hours he had no interest in answering my fawning questions any further. He thanked me and left the room, ready to move on. Sadly, Ella passed away several days later. Martin gathered the family together, buried his wife, and didn't linger in his past. He moved back to Chicago to be near his children and grandchildren and renewed his role as the patriarch of the family—no longer just as a husband and a father. From a life that I imagined would be wrapping up and fading away after such a loss, he quietly and resolutely entered an encore phase as the leader of the family. Without him, the family lacked the cohesion and direction that made it thrive.

Unfortunately, we lose greatly when we cannot see the immense achievements and potential that people have in later life. Such energy is usually there and quite active, but we too often fail to pay attention to it, revel in its role in our life, and feel gratitude for its existence. When we denigrate aging and only see it primarily as a time of decline and weakness, we rob ourselves of one of the most influential and powerful forces in our life. The antidote is simple: look at aging people and ask about their reserve, learn about their resilience, and marvel at their ability to renew and reinvent themselves. When you see and experience these forces—as an observer and as a participant—it changes the way you view aging. It gives aging a pulse and a direction. It shows us a wide and diverse culture of aging—in full-bodied form and color—that is worthy of great celebration.

The Culture of Age

When I was a twenty-one-year-old college student, I had the extraordinary opportunity to meet a famous psychiatrist by the name of Henry A. Murray, who was one of the greatest scholars on the human personality. During my visits, Murray taught me a profound lesson about how and why aging gives us the ability to thrive. Murray was ninety-three at the time and appeared as a robust, gray-bearded sage sitting in a wheelchair. He lived in a well-kept, book-filled Victorian house tucked away in a quiet and shady neighborhood several blocks from Harvard's massive psychology tower. I was introduced to Murray by his equally long-bearded assistant, Eugene Taylor, who resembled in form and figure his icon and research subject—the great American psychologist William James. Murray had been a friend of Carl Jung and an acquaintance of Sigmund Freud, and was renowned himself as the former director of the Harvard Psychological Clinic and the creator of the thematic apperception test, or TAT, one of the most widely used projective tests aside from the Rorschach ink blots. Murray was also known for helping to develop the psychological profiling system used by the Office of Strategic Services during World War II, which later became the Central Intelligence Agency. As one might imagine, stepping into Murray's house was a journey back in time in which I felt surrounded by the powerful and transcendent voices of those who founded the very field to which I was devoting my life.

During one of my visits, I sat upstairs in his study and found myself intrigued by the bric-a-brac on his desk, including several intricately carved ivory whale's teeth, or scrimshaw. When I asked him why he had collected so many of these relics, Murray informed me that he was a devotee and part-time scholar of Herman Melville, the great American author of *Moby-Dick* and *Billy Budd*, which were both set on whaling ships. He loved how Melville wrote some of the richest literary descriptions of various personalities. He then showed me a bronze medallion that he had commissioned as the unofficial "coat of arms" for the Harvard Psychological Clinic. It was engraved with the images of several sea creatures swimming beneath the placid expression of a human face. To Murray, the image on the medallion was the perfect graphic metaphor for the human personality, with our superficial appearance lying above all the dynamic forces below. The medallion also bore a quote from the apocryphal Gospel of Thomas, which read:

> Let not him who seeks cease until he finds,
> And when he finds he shall be astonished.

The quote captured Murray's belief that one must delve into the study of a person without prejudice or hesitation, searching for the great variety and depths of human expression. The reward will be a full and astonishing vision of our current and potential personality. Murray wrote that each personality was a "full Congress of orators and pressure-groups, of children, demagogues, communists, isolationists, war-mongers, mugwumps, grafters, log-rollers, lobbyists, Caesars and Christs, Machiavellis and Judases, Tories and Promethean revolutionists. And a psychologist who does not know this in himself, whose mind is locked against the flux of images and feelings, should be encouraged to make friends . . . with the various members of his household."

This image stuck with me permanently after my encounters with Murray: the individual person as a congress of many. As I later began to work as a doctor, I kept this detailed view of each patient in my mind and applied it to every encounter. We see a single face and hear a simple story, but that is only a view of the surface. Beneath each exterior and within each person is a vast repository of knowledge, skills, experiences, eyewitness accounts, thoughts, feelings, and passions that move like Murray's great leviathans through countless oceans. When I first began working with aged individuals, I didn't know whether this perspective would apply. Were the halls of the congress emptying out? Were the seas drying up? As I delved into my work, I saw the opposite and I fully realized the power of Murray's approach. Aging was filling each human congress with more and more personas and passions. The sea was richer and more diverse. Aging banged the gavel and brought the session into heated discussion and debate. Aging moved the great currents from sea bottom to surface and from shore to shore. Aging kept life flowing.

There is an imperative, then, to view ourselves in our totality. Put together, the accumulating products of our aging self represent a rich tapestry of abilities, interests, experiences, relationships, and commitments that can be described as our *age culture*. The term *culture* can be defined in several ways. On a small scale, it is both the nutrient-rich medium and the act that promotes the growth of a life form. We use *cultures* or we *culture* yeast, bacteria, or cell lines to learn or create something much greater. On a large scale, *culture* refers to the collective rituals, customs, behaviors, and arts of a cohesive group. The term *age culture* brings these two meanings together. On an individual level, it is composed of all our abilities and experiences; on an interpersonal level, it represents our dynamic presence and connections with others; on a family or community level, it is expressed in the collective activities and attitudes of aging individuals.

If you want to understand your own age culture, ask yourself the following questions:

Who was I? What have I learned, accomplished, and experienced in my past? What are my essential skills and expertise? The answers represent your reserves of wisdom.

Who am I? What do I spend most of my time doing or who do I spend most of my time with? What are my current activities and passions? The answers show you what your purpose in life is.

Who will I be? What do I want to do, see, and experience in the future? With whom do I want to spend my time? What do I want to leave behind for others? The answers tell you how you can renew or reinvent yourself.

Your age culture is a growth medium for your life. It has a nutrient-rich base, a bubbling process of coping and adjusting to change, and a rich froth of new activity. The optimal recognition and construction of an age culture can end the constricted notion of old age that we have for too long seen as our inevitable fate. It is at this point that we can experience true liberation and authenticity and finally be able to *say what we want to say*. The true elixir of aging that lies behind all these endeavors is *creativity*—brewing and bubbling with each year, impervious to physical decline and even resistant to cognitive impairment in the ninth stage.

Thriving in the Ninth Stage

Most schemes of aging leave out those individuals in the ninth stage who have significant cognitive and/or physical impairment. It is still possible to thrive in the ninth stage, but doing so requires the help of others and a determination to work around barriers and identify the best approaches. Engagement in the arts is one of the most fruitful avenues here, since our ability to enjoy the world through our senses is persistent even in the most severe physical or mental conditions.

◌ʀ

I have known and admired Celia for many years, because she is the mother of my close friend Mariana. Over the past fifteen years, I have watched Celia age and struggle with the loss of her husband and then the progressive development of Parkinson's disease. At age eighty-five, she is facing several daunting challenges. The Parkinson's disease has slowed her movements considerably and she is unable or reluctant to do most of the routine activities she once enjoyed such as shopping, exercising, and traveling. The Parkinson's has also brought with it the associated challenges of depression, apathy, and mild cognitive impairment. Everything about her is slower, less engaged, and even resistant. This has been difficult for Mariana to watch, since she is used to having a mom who is a brilliant architect, an insightful conversationalist, an astute shopping companion, and a wise grandmother for her three children.

Nonetheless, Mariana has fought the apathy and resistance tooth and nail. When she first noticed her mother's slowing movements, she brought her to a neurologist for comprehensive evaluation and treatment. In addition to medication, she enrolled Celia in physical therapy three times a week and brought in a massage therapist. For Celia's depression, Mariana consulted a psychiatrist and brought in a talk therapist who would come to her apartment and speak to her in her native language of Portuguese. She also brought her mother to drawing and music classes, a cooking class, a computer class, and countless family gatherings. Celia usually goes along with Mariana and has glimmers of interest and enjoyment, but they fade quickly. Sometimes she simply refuses Mariana's plans and expresses complete disinterest.

Celia's situation is complex and challenging. Parkinson's disease is a progressive neurologic condition whereby the degeneration of a small bundle of cells in the brain leads to slowed movements, a shuffling gait, a masked facial expression, tremors, and periods of almost complete freezing. Medications can temporary liberate movements but also cause side effects, such as hallucinations and paranoia. It is common for individuals with Parkinson's to develop depression and dementia as well. Whereas these effects are obvious, there are more insidious changes that I suspect affect Celia deeply: a fear or even terror of falling, embarrassment in social gatherings, a lack of energy and motivation for activities, and a loss of morale and dignity. Mariana has been doing her best for her mom, but the battle is tough.

One day, however, Mariana made an amazing discovery. Celia had reluctantly agreed to accompany the family to an out-of-town wedding at a resort hotel. On the afternoon after the ceremony, everyone was lounging around the pool and listening to some lively merengue music. Mariana was shocked to see her mother suddenly stand up and stride across part of the outdoor patio, swaying in rhythm to the music. She was dancing! It was almost an unconscious act, but Mariana seemed lost in a happy revelry. Upon their return to Miami, Mariana hatched a plan. She knew of a woman named Diosiris who taught a Zumba class to seniors, and begged her to consider giving a private class in Celia's apartment. Diosiris is used to such requests, and is eager to help since she has seen the transformations in so many aging individuals who start off rejecting Zumba. "I can't do it," they tell her, "it's for young people." Diosiris knows better. She teaches a special class for aging individuals that combines dance and music to improve mobility, strength, and balance and instill confidence. If a person can stand or sit, or use a walker or a wheelchair, he or she can be taught Zumba.

Diosiris even works with blind individuals who can't see what she does but can hear and feel the beat of the music through the air and from the floors. It is an infectious combination—happy and smiling instructors wearing beaded and belled body wraps and dancing to salsa, merengue, Cumbia, and reggaeton music. The classes that Diosiris teaches are her passion, and she learned its benefits firsthand shortly after she moved to Miami from Barranquilla, Colombia. After she had her first child, she was struggling with adjusting to her new country and was depressed and overweight. Zumba was a liberation; it reminded her of her dance career back in Colombia and made her feel healthy and happy.

Celia was reluctant to try Zumba, but she lit up during and after each class, and for a few hours her movements became more fluid, and she was more animated and engaged in conversation. Normally, it is a struggle to get Celia to do one thing a day; after Zumba, this average moved up to two. It's not a cure, but it's certainly a reinvention of Celia into a more active and sociable person after many years of struggle. This transformation, limited as it may be, illustrates three key points of creative aging in the ninth stage. First, it requires the help and creativity of others. Second, it involves a lot of trial and error. Third, it reminds us that there are always avenues of engagement that can be tapped into despite significant physical and mental disabilities. Music, dance, and the visual arts are several particularly powerful examples. We can all hearken to the wise and poetic words of writer Diane Ackerman: "A bell with a crack in it may not ring as clearly, but it can ring as sweetly."

PART IV

The Action Plan

I have needed all that time to reach the stage where I can say what I want to say.

—HENRI MATISSE

Chapter 7

Redefining and Re-Aging

IF YOU ASK long-lived people what their secret to life is, you will get a diverse and highly personalized range of answers. Some of these responses may apply to your own life; some may seem strange or even counterintuitive. The bottom line is that *you* have to determine your own meaningful path, built upon your unique age-given strengths of wisdom, purpose, and creativity. No one can do it for you. This action plan will help you identify, develop, and optimize these age-given strengths and appreciate your own age culture. The ultimate goal is not only to live longer but to live a better, more purposeful life. This action plan can be applied to every aging person, but will need to be adjusted based on the context in which you see yourself or someone in the ninth stage whom you are trying to help:

I'm good: If you generally consider yourself to be healthy and happy, the action plan will highlight your achievements and abilities, prepare you for potential adversity, and inspire you to expand or pursue new, creative endeavors.

I'm stuck: If you are struggling with physical or mental problems and feel slowed down or even stuck in a geropause, the action plan will provide a roadmap to move forward. Keep in mind, however, that you can't always make changes alone, but must engage the help of family, friends, and professionals. Having to depend on others is not only practical but healthy, since it builds connections with others and opens up opportunities to give back. This book was directly inspired by many similarly challenged and stuck individuals who taught me key lessons about resilience and creativity!

I need help: For those individuals in the ninth stage, the action plan will provide their caregivers, family members, friends, clinicians, and others with a structure to understand and value their age culture along with practical strategies to get them more engaged in enjoyable and meaningful activities. Ultimately, these exercises show us the value, dignity, and sanctity of our aging selves.

The action plan is simple and requires a few hours of your time. Besides this book, you need nothing other than several sheets of paper and a pen or pencil. It requires that you have an open mind, a willingness to examine your life, and perhaps a few trusted people to provide input. The action plan consists of five basic steps:

1. **Reserve**
   Define your reserve. This step will help you fully appreciate the scope of your wisdom.
2. **Resilience**
   Examine your resilience. This step will highlight your purpose in life.
3. **Reinvention**
   Consider pathways for renewal and reinvention. This step will identify potential barriers to change, light up your age culture, and spark your creativity.

4. Legacy

Consider your legacy. What do you want to leave behind for others and for the future? The answers may prompt important decisions or creative endeavors.

5. Celebration

Plan a ritual or ceremony to celebrate your aging. We have rituals and ceremonies for every major transition in life, but not aging. Now that you've reexamined your own aging in a positive light, find a way to celebrate it.

I hope that this book has already helped you to redefine how you look at aging. I hope that this action plan will help you age better by improving how you value the aging process, guide yourself through stress, and find ways to creatively address change. We are trying again and again to make life better even as we may want it to be longer. I call this process *re-aging* because it is built upon so many factors and actions that begin with the prefix *re*. In essence, we have the ever-present opportunity to revise and redo our aging process to bring the best possible experience and outcome.

My Miami Cabinet Tries It Out

Over the years, I have introduced every element of this action plan to patients, caregivers, and interested groups in both formal and informal ways during therapy sessions, discussions, or lectures. Once I compiled a structured plan for this book, however, I decided to do a complete test run with a group of aged individuals that I call my "Miami cabinet." The group was actually put together by my friend Judy, who happens to be the vice mayor of a small oceanside community north of Miami. My instructions were simple: find a diverse group of individuals in their seventies, eighties, and nineties who would like to talk about aging. The group came together one sunny afternoon around the dining table at Judy's house, plied with deli sandwiches, pickles, bottles of seltzer, and a dessert platter overflowing with rugelach and black-and-white cookies. We were ready to begin.

My cabinet was a lively group who filled our session from start to finish with life stories and tales, anecdotes, jokes, and wise aphorisms. I was blown away. I imagined that I would have to educate them about all I had learned about aging from years of study and clinical work, but they schooled me quicker than I could get the words out of my mouth. It was as if they walked off the pages of this book and showed me in vivid detail all the strengths of aging. I was humbled, impressed, and inspired. I wanted every doubter and castigator of aging to be sitting there, listening to this group and realizing their immense value to their families and the wider community. Their stories and wisdom will illuminate each step of the action plan.

Shirley is an 80-year-old widowed woman. I featured part of her story earlier in the book when talking about resilience.

Ken is a 78-year-old single man who works as a facility manager.

David is an 87-year-old navy veteran who had multiple careers and is now an author and playwright.

Peter is a 90-year-old World War II veteran who is now a retired real estate broker.

Alfred is a 92-year-old World War II veteran who worked as an electrical contractor in New York.

Sydell is an 89-year-old married woman from Brooklyn and has been Alfred's wife for the past 68 years.

In addition to this group, there were several individuals who could not attend the meeting at Judy's house, but still participated in elements of the action plan:

Jim is a 75-year-old divorced man from Wisconsin who works as a chauffeur.

Norma is a 90-year-old widowed woman from Barbados, West Indies.

Step 1: Reserve

Define your reserve. We begin our action plan by defining our current reserve of wisdom based on the five types of wise people and their various roles: savant, sage, curator, creator, and seer. Detailed descriptions of each type can be found in "The Crown of Wisdom" table at the end of Chapter 2. Review these descriptions and then create your own table on a sheet of paper in which you record your reserves of wisdom, based on the Defining Your Reserve template on page 164. Imagine everything that you have done and can do now, as if you are preparing a life resume. Consider this an opportunity to brag. No addition is too trivial. You might want to ask someone who knows you well to review it and suggest additions. If you are filling this out for someone else, tally his or her lifetime of experience and knowledge. This exercise primarily answers the questions of "who was I?" and "who am I now?" that will be helpful when revealing your age culture in Step 3.

During my meeting with the Miami cabinet, David was eager to talk about his wisdom since he had done so much in his eighty-seven years. His life story was fascinating. He grew up in the small town of Montague on the eastern shore of Lake Michigan, hailing from a family that can trace its lineage back to the first settlers in Michigan and a great-great-great-grandfather who was a soldier in the Revolutionary War. David opened up the group discussion with a summary of his life: "I'm a person who has lived nine decades and has done all those things I wanted to do and have no regrets. As a young person, I dreamed of living in various parts of the world,

Defining Your Reserve

WISDOM	YOUR RESERVE, ROLES, AND WISDOM
SAVANT: Core knowledge, experiences, skills, and interests	
SAGE: Key influence and decision-making roles. Key values (e.g., important beliefs, ethics, and morals) and virtues (e.g., personal characteristics) that you put into action	
CURATOR: Social and community interests and involvement	
CREATOR: Creative activities, roles, or interests	
SEER: Spiritual, religious, or philosophical interests, perspectives, or pursuits	

having romances, and writing about my life, and I have done everything. I put the world together the way I wanted. I can go at any time." In his chart, David outlined his many careers and skills.

David was a tall and impeccably dressed man who swept into the room with a debonair style. He exuded pride and confidence and was not shy to outline his past and ongoing interests and accomplishments. It was difficult to believe that he was eighty-seven years old. He has always had a romantic partner and never wanted to have children. His current partner is a thirty-two-year-old soccer player, and when one friend stated that "either he is really into you or he is the best actor," David retorted, "Who cares!" There is an ageless quality to David's current abilities and lifestyle, and I view him as a superager whose cognitive skills seem to have hardly declined. He is

David's Chart of Wisdom

SAVANT: Core knowledge, experiences, skills, and interests	I have had six careers: (1) gardener; (2) naval officer who witnessed the testing of the hydrogen bomb on Bikini Atoll in 1952–53; (3) advertising executive; (4) ballet dancer and then manager of the Joffrey Ballet; (5) creative director for cosmetic companies Revlon and L'Oréal; (6) author and playwright.
SAGE: Key influence and decision-making roles. Key values (e.g., important beliefs, ethics, and morals) and virtues (e.g., personal characteristics) that you put into action	Producing a play requires constant negotiating and organizing. I am confident in my creative vision and decision making and fearless about letting others know about my preferences.
CURATOR: Social and community interests and involvement	My books and plays allow me to reach out to the community and teach them about my perspectives.
CREATOR: Creative activities, roles, or interests	I am currently writing books and plays, including one that was just staged in London. I am the author of over 30 books, including *How to Hit 70 Doing 100*.
SEER: Spiritual, religious, or philosophical interests, perspectives, or pursuits	My worldview is not religious per se but is optimistic and accepting. I would sum up my life perspectives this way: Everything I expected to happen didn't happen and a lot of terrible things happened that no one expected. Also: Failing and succeeding are the same thing as long as you try.

as active at eighty-seven as he was at seventy. David has constantly reinvented himself in life as his burgeoning experience and creativity has been supported by tremendous energy and enthusiasm.

Sydell is nearly the same age as David and has equal amounts of energy, but her roles are different in that they are primarily family-based.

Sydell's Chart of Wisdom

SAVANT: Core knowledge, experiences, skills, and interests	I see my current role as the matriarch of a family of 5 children ages 59 thru 67, 12 grandchildren, and 7 great-grandchildren with 2 on the way. I am proud that I have always had a job, dating back to my first one paying 12.5 cents an hour working in a dance studio.
SAGE: Key influence and decision-making roles. Key values (e.g., important beliefs, ethics, and morals) and virtues (e.g., personal characteristics) that you put into action	I am a devoted wife and caregiver for my husband, Alfred. I have guided him through 2 bouts of cancer. I feel like I am the emotional lead for my family. I always communicate my feelings to my kids—that is my legacy. For many years, I was the commissioner of a youth athletic program and worked to get young people involved in sports and team play.
CURATOR: Social and community interests and involvement	I see my daily involvement as a curator since I am always there for everyone. My main role has been as a volunteer worker for a polling station during elections and as an unpaid bookkeeper for a mobile home park.
CREATOR: Creative activities, roles, or interests	I often have to problem-solve issues that come up with my husband, children, and grandchildren.
SEER: Spiritual, religious, or philosophical interests, perspectives, or pursuits	I am Jewish and attend religious services occasionally and celebrate major Jewish holidays. My two mottos are: I have to wake up with a smile on my face; and I am busy as a bee.

Sydell embodies the term *matriarch* in that she continues to run her family of sixty-eight years, including her husband, Alfred. At first, Alfred was reluctant to fill out his wisdom chart, with Sydell chiming in and trying to define it for him. Despite her benevolent intrusions, however, Alfred held his ground and had a lot to say about several key experiences in his life that revealed him to be a dedicated and altruistic man. As a young ensign on the destroyer escort ship USS *Coolbaugh* during World War II, Alfred recalled helping to save ninety-one injured and burned sailors who had jumped off the aircraft escort USS *Suwanee* after it was struck by a Japanese kamikaze pilot in 1944. Later in the war, he remembered seeing the iconic raising of the American flag on Mount Suribachi during the battle for the island of Iwo Jima. In his later career as an electrician, one of his proudest jobs was fixing the electrical system in the Statue of Liberty. For his large family, Alfred is a seer who projects steadiness and contentment: "I don't think about aging. I enjoy every day and age doesn't come into it."

Norma is ninety years old and grew up on the island of Barbados. In 1925, when she was only a year old, her ship captain father was lost at sea when his schooner disappeared during a major storm. Norma was an amateur dancer and actress as a young woman. She was married for fifty-three years and had three children; her five grandchildren include one who is a famous professional dancer and actress. She survived Hurricane Hugo in 1989, huddling with her family for hours in a 3-foot-deep storm surge after the roof blew off their house. Norma lost her only son in 1999 and her husband in 2003. In some ways, she currently represents someone in the ninth stage, as she suffers from significant arthritic joint pain and immobility, facial pain from postherpetic neuralgia, hearing loss, memory loss, apathy, and a kidney packed with stones. Norma mourns her loss of independence. "She is living on a slippery slope" describes her daughter Margaret, who moved her into her home in Miami to keep a closer eye on her. Despite these struggles, Norma retains a healthy reserve of multiple points of wisdom and roles (see page 168).

I saw and tasted Norma's wisdom firsthand when she and her daughter brought me an aromatic and tasty black brick of Barbados Great Cake during the recent winter holidays. This liquor-soaked

Norma's Chart of Wisdom
(prepared by her daughter Margaret)

SAVANT: Core knowledge, experiences, skills, and interests	Norma was a tap dancer and an actress. She is a survivor of a major hurricane. She has dealt with the losses of her son and husband. Norma loves to play Scrabble and work word jumbles on the computer. She has a great sense of humor. She is an expert at making Barbados Great Cake.
SAGE: Key influence and decision-making roles. Key values (e.g., important beliefs, ethics, and morals) and virtues (e.g., personal characteristics) that you put into action	Norma is the matriarch of her family, and her children and grandchildren still seek her guidance.
CURATOR: Social and community interests and involvement	Norma is involved in her Methodist church. Her personality attracts people; they just love her. When she sees someone at church who appears to not be doing well, she will actively approach him or her and say, "You don't look yourself today. What's up?"
CREATOR: Creative activities, roles, or interests	Norma has an amazing ability to create acrostic poems, and the pastor at her church has asked her to create one for each new member and for every newly married couple.
SEER: Spiritual, religious, or philosophical interests, perspectives, or pursuits	Norma has a strong faith in God. She prays a lot, meditates every day, and reads religious texts extensively.

delight, also known as Bajan Black Cake, is the Caribbean version of British plum pudding and is traditionally served at Christmas-time and weddings on the island. Three months before the cake is baked, Norma begins the process of grinding up a combination of raisins, prunes, currants, and citron and then soaking the paste in a brew of wine, Mount Gay Rum, and an alcoholic syrup called falernum. Margaret has learned from the master how to mix in countless eggs, sift the flour, and then fold in the soaked and minced fruit along with brown sugar, butter, chopped cherries and almonds, and lemon and vanilla extract. The cake is baked and then soaked in more Barbados rum before an icing of almond paste is applied. Norma was thrilled to present my team and me with a chunk of her culinary handiwork, and she smiled and chortled in delight upon hearing how much it was enjoyed. As the years have gone by, Margaret assumes more of the heavy lifting of both the preparation and creation of the cake, but Norma earns and enjoys a lion's share of pride in the process.

As you can see from the wisdom charts of David, Sydell, and Norma, it is relatively easy to fill up the various forms of wisdom once you review your life accomplishments and interests. The chart should bring a sense of pride along with ideas of what one can still do. Your chart will be reviewed again and built upon in Step 3.

Step 2: Resilience

Examine your resilience. The goal of Step 2 is to review one or more major age points in your life so as to extract and boost your modes of resilient coping. It will identify your main supports, adaptive behaviors, and key resources. This process will highlight your age-related purpose in life. It is likely that you are not in an age point during the course of this exercise, and so you will have to select the most recent stressful situation that will suffice. The age points of Judy and Jim from our Miami cabinet will illustrate this process well. You can draw your own age point grid on a sheet of paper (with larger boxes for each category than appear in this template) and fill it in as you recall and evaluate the age point.

The Age Point Grid

EVENTS:	
SUSPENSION:	
RECKONING:	
RESOLUTION:	

My friend Judy, the organizer of the Miami cabinet, came to me several years ago in the throes of a critical age point. I first met Judy when she brought her husband to my office for an evaluation. He had been suffering from Alzheimer's disease for years and needed round-the-clock care and supervision for dressing, feeding, and dealing with agitated behaviors. He was relatively calm and stable at that stage and only needed a few minor medication adjustments. Everything seemed on track for the next year, until I got a desperate call from Judy at my home one Sunday evening. I could barely hear her voice over the phone, as she was trembling and crying. She had fallen into an acute state of panic and depression, convinced that she had a terminal illness after learning that her liver enzymes were elevated on a routine blood test. As her emotional state deteriorated, she withdrew into her bed and cowered under the covers. Even though she did not yet have any diagnosis or even clear indication of a serious illness, the very idea that she could die, leaving her husband and son without her care, was enough to pull the legs from under her. "I felt like one foot was in the grave and the other was on a banana peel," she told me. This was a relatively precipitous fall into an age point, triggered no doubt by perpetual caregiver burden, exhaustion, and worries about balancing her political responsibilities with being both a wife and a mom. Her initial age point grid appears here:

Judy's Age Point Grid: Events and Suspension

EVENTS: Routine blood tests indicate elevated liver enzymes and possible liver disease.
SUSPENSION: Shock and worry that the test results may indicate a terminal illness. Terrible anxiety and panic, crying, feelings of despair, and loss of energy, interest, and appetite. I hid in my room and pulled the covers over my head.
RECKONING:
RESOLUTION:

I was surprised by Judy's call, as she had been one of the brightest, calmest, and most organized caregivers I had ever met. The blood tests did not seem alarming to me and did not, at that point, indicate anything serious or even terminal—but that was beside the point. They symbolized an existential threat to Judy, who counted upon her health to care for her husband and son. I met with her immediately to understand these emotional currents and to provide some relief with some counseling and, given the paralyzing intensity of her emotions, a short-acting tranquilizer. The medication would at least allow her to get out of her house, eat, and resume some of her daily responsibilities while a longer-lasting antidepressant and ongoing talk therapy had time to work. Once Judy was calmer, the reckoning could begin.

Judy's self-image and confidence had already been weakened by the rigors of caregiving, so the relatively minor news of a potential medical problem seemed like a death sentence to her. Every one of her fears took center stage and overwhelmed her. For the first time in her life, she had to face the previously foreign and unacceptable idea that she was mortal and would, at some point, have to rely on others for help. Fortunately, she dragged herself into my office and

Judy's Age Point Grid, Continued: Reckoning

EVENTS: Routine blood tests indicate elevated liver enzymes and possible liver disease.
SUSPENSION: Shock and worry that the test results may indicate a terminal illness. Terrible anxiety and panic, crying, feelings of despair, and loss of energy, interest, and appetite. I hid in my room and pulled the covers over my head.
RECKONING: I need to care for my husband, but who will take my place if I am disabled or dead? My son needs my guidance and support, and will be essentially orphaned if I die. I have always been a stable and independent person, but I now feel out of control. I have seen myself as young and capable, but now I feel old and weak.
RESOLUTION:

began the process of healing. The medications and reassurance worked well enough to calm Judy and get her back on track, but it wasn't until further blood tests ruled out any serious disease that the cloud lifted. The resolution was not simply returning to her baseline. She learned several deep lessons about herself and her life that inoculated her to a certain extent against further crises.

Judy was a changed person after this age point, and it clarified her purpose in life as a caregiver for her husband, a guide for her adult son, and a dedicated politician in her community. She was able to plunge back into all three roles with renewed energy and deepened compassion. She also took on a new role as my unofficial ambassador and big sister for several other ailing caregivers at our memory center. Judy formed a close circle of friends with several of these individuals and helped start a support group with them. Her age point was a brief period of agony, but it sharpened and expanded her purpose in life. Every time we see each other, we reference that crisis and marvel at how it transformed the caregiver support program in our memory center.

Judy's Age Point Grid Completed: Resolution

EVENTS: Routine blood tests indicate elevated liver enzymes and possible liver disease.
SUSPENSION: Shock and worry that the test results may indicate a terminal illness. Terrible anxiety and panic, crying, feeling of despair, and loss of energy, interest, and appetite. I hid in my room and pulled the covers over my head.
RECKONING: I need to care for my husband, but who will take my place if I am disabled or dead? My son needs my guidance and support, and will be essentially orphaned if I die. I have always been a stable and independent person, but I now feel out of control. I have seen myself as young and capable, but now I feel old and weak.
RESOLUTION: I am not dying, and I now realize that when I face medical situations I need to remain calm and think logically about the situation. My emotional Achilles' heel is my concern for my son. Anything that seems to threaten my ability to be his mother may precipitate significant anxiety. I feel more compassion for others with medical problems, and realize how important it is to reach out for help and to be a support for others.

In contrast to Judy, other individuals have age points that consist of multiple stresses. This was the case with my friend Jim, who is the driver for one of my patients. He is a seventy-five-year-old divorced father of two sons and three grandchildren who grew up in the North Woods of Wisconsin, where his grandparents ran a fishing resort. He was an avid racquetball player who traveled the country for tournaments, and worked as a manager for athletic clubs until he reinvented himself as a limousine driver in his mid-fifties. Jim remains a committed athlete and sports fan, and is a particularly diehard fan of both the Wisconsin Badgers and the Green Bay Packers. In fact, Jim and I initially struck up a conversation about our love for the Packers after I confessed my Cheese-head roots to him and he invited me to a raucous Packers sports bar in Fort Lauderdale.

Jim has faced numerous major stresses, including a diagnosis of tongue cancer, severe illness in a close family member, and the divorce of each of his sons. These events have been difficult for him, but Jim's age point suspension for each one has been muted by skills he has learned from previous health crises, including quadruple bypass surgery, atrial fibrillation, and stage 3 cancer of his tonsil. When he learned about his most recent cancer diagnosis, he was worried but took the attitude of "Let's fix this and move on. I won't lose any sleep over it. I have a problem and there's a solution." During the reckoning phase, he wrestled with the possibility of having speech and swallowing problems, but tried to keep an optimistic mind-set: "I just felt I would be okay. I never worried about the treatment not working." In fact, Jim told me that he gets more worked up during the average Packers game! That might sound like an exaggeration, but it gives him a yardstick of acute distress that he can use to help downplay other worries. Jim continues to have occasional, painful emotional reminders—call them brief returns to the suspension stage of his age point—but each time he returns to the well-worn pathways employed in the reckoning and resolution phases to get through them. When these falter a bit, he reaches out to trusted family and friends either to talk it out or to simply feel comforted in their presence. In the end, this process works just fine. We can summarize Jim's age point in the grid on page 175.

Not surprising, Jim is a dear friend, father, and fellow athlete to many. The other bowlers in his league are, on average, twenty to thirty years younger, and can't believe that Jim is the age of most of their fathers. Aging has brought a multitude of medical and family stresses to Jim, but it has also helped him develop much wisdom, an incredibly positive attitude, and several undying points of purpose through work, love of family, and sports.

Jim's Age Point Grid

EVENTS: Getting a diagnosis of tongue cancer. In the same year, I learned about a serious illness in a family member and of the pending divorces of my two sons.

SUSPENSION: Mild nervousness but I take a positive approach: "It will be OK." "There is a problem and it has a solution." "I worry more during a Packers game. I can handle the stress."

RECKONING: How will I deal with possible speech and swallowing problems? I am slightly concerned about being able to continue working. I wonder how my sons will cope with their divorces.

RESOLUTION: I got a second opinion and found a surgeon to perform my surgery using a robotic system, which significantly reduced recovery time and side effects. I am fully recovered and not bothered by a mild speech impediment. I continue to be a support for my sons, a reliable driver for my clients, a regular bowler in a league, and a Badgers and Packers fan (or fanatic) to the end.

In constructing your own age point grid, then, consider how both Judy and Jim faced stresses that were both real and symbolic. Don't feel as if you have to analyze a major calamity. Just pick some event that challenged your coping skills; created some emotional upset; caused you to question your goals, beliefs, or values; and then, hopefully, led to a resolution for the problem but also an expanded notion of your purpose in life. Sometimes an issue that you want to avoid, or didn't think of due to unconscious resistance, may actually be the perfect age point to analyze. If you find yourself stuck in one of the stages of an age point, consider this an opportunity for growth. Examine how others may have moved forward. Consult with a trusted family member or friend who can provide some perspective. Do not be afraid to reach out to a professional for help. Remember that aging has given you a multitude of strengths to move forward. The end result can make all the difference.

Step 3: Reinvention

Consider pathways for renewal and reinvention. The purpose of this exercise is to reenergize your most important values and pursuits and explore ways to reinvent yourself in the face of age-related changes in your life circumstances. Here you will identify potential barriers to change, recognize your own age culture, and commit yourself to *age imperatives* composed of creative and meaningful activities, relationships, and pursuits. The good news is that the previous exercises have already prepared you for this third step. It will also help guide the development of vital and enjoyable life activities and connections for individuals in the ninth stage.

At this point, you might meet immediate resistance that effectively says, "I can't change" (or "The person can't change"). These include some of the following conditions:

- Physical problems (e.g., "I'm not able" or "It hurts too much.")
- Emotional problems (e.g., "I don't feel well enough to do it.")
- Negative attitudes (e.g., "I don't want to.")
- Lack of resources (e.g., "I can't pay for it" or "I can't get rides.")
- Lack of permission (e.g., "My spouse won't allow it.")

These barriers might limit or even prevent a single activity or may fuel an entire geropause. Regardless, it is still possible to move forward by finding work-arounds, even in the ninth stage. If you feel stuck, keep in mind that there is always potential for immense change in late life. You just have to recognize your strengths and move forward. Creative aging is not only life changing but life affirming. It doesn't merely steer the ship of age and keep it away from dangerous shoals, but finds new currents of water and wind and innovative shapes of sails and rudders to carry you beyond where you've gone before.

Let's begin by identifying the incredibly diverse accomplishments and strengths that aging has brought you—what I am calling your *age culture*. Think deeply and broadly about all your interests, abilities, experiences, skills, and values. Review your wisdom chart and age point grids. Take a sheet of paper and create a grid similar to that for "Your Age Culture" here:

Your Age Culture

WHO I WAS	WHO I AM
WHO I WILL BE	MY LEGACY

To fill in the grid, ask yourself the following questions:

Who was I? What elements defined my past self?

Who am I? What elements still define me and occupy the most time in my life?

Who will I be? As I age, what elements do I want to retain, expand upon, or change? How will I do that?

What is my legacy? What do I want to leave behind for others? (This question will be discussed in Step 4.)

Be generous to yourself when filling in your age culture grid. It's okay to brag. Don't worry about what is necessarily attainable, but dream a little. The point of defining your age culture here is to emphasize all your strengths and to begin the process of redefining your aging self. By looking at who you were in the past, who you are now in the present, and who you would like to be in the future, you are integrating your purpose with a positive view of the future. In her wonderful book *Agewise*, Margaret Morganroth Gullette emphasizes that it is critically important to see ourself as actively growing with age, as opposed to falling prey to the prevailing narrative of aging as only a time of decline.

When Matisse began reinventing himself as a master of paper cutouts instead of a painter on canvas, he worked on a book called *Jazz*. The title is a good analogy for the freedom of rhythm and movement that you want to seek with age, what a biographer of his described as "vital and free . . . constantly alternating between risk and success, mischance and luck." Some people are exuberant to the point of carelessness in this regard, acting like Matisse's artistic portrayal of the mythical Icarus, who donned a suit of feathers but flew too close to the sun, only to realize the perils of his hubris as he was plunging to the enveloping sea below. Take a lesson on aging from the same story and think more like Icarus's father, Daedalus, the creator of the wings, the careful guide and admonisher of a youthful, foolish son who didn't head his warnings. Dream, but take care. Tally your deficits and barriers, but lead with your strengths.

Of all members of the Miami cabinet, Ken was the most concise in describing himself. His philosophy of life was simple and straightforward: "I avoid doctors and churches. I treat you like I want to be treated." Aging? "I don't think much about it." One might be misled by Ken's paucity of words, but once I got him talking, his age culture burst open.

Ken's age culture reveals a proud, hardworking man with a fascinating past, a creative spirit, and total dedication to his work. If

Ken's Age Culture

WHO I WAS	WHO I AM
• African American, born in Virginia • Became a car salesman to earn money and get a car • Started a commercial cleaning business, then sold it • Became the only African American in town on the Chamber of Commerce • Moved to New York and worked for ABC to vet prizefights. Traveled around the world. • Knew Muhammed Ali • Lost my girlfriend of 17 years in 2003	• Dedicated facilities director for an oceanside community • Never missed a day of work in last 15 years • Follow the Golden Rule: "I treat you like I want to be treated" • Avoid doctors due to their tendency to order too many time-consuming, unnecessary tests • Avoid churches because of their past role in segregation • My family is the oceanside community that I work for.
WHO I WILL BE • I plan to work until I can't. • Retirement is not a word in my vocabulary.	**MY LEGACY** Total support and dedication for the community. The entire group at the table knows my loyalty and expertise. I help the community function.

his age culture were a financial portfolio, it would be doing great with one notable deficiency—it has no insurance for the future. Ken's life is his work. His work is his family. I imagine him working up to the day he dies. I base this on a story Ken told about having to go into the hospital to take several tests. After several days, he felt that the doctor was taking too much time to reach a diagnosis and make a definitive plan. Refusing to wait another minute, Ken took off his hospital gown and walked out. Later that day, he went right back to work. As foolhardy as that might sound if something truly serious was brewing, it illustrates Ken's ultimate strength: a total dedication to a singular purpose in his life, in which he is incredibly successful. The other members at the table fell all over one another to praise Ken's role in the community. He is like the wizard behind the curtain of the community, keeping everything clean, well maintained, and running smoothly.

Once you create your age culture, you will have a keen view of your overall value to yourself and others, a stronger belief in your ability to accomplish things (i.e., your self-efficacy), and a glance into your own future. In Step 4 we will talk more about legacy. At this stage, you can use your age culture to think about what you want your aged life to be. The choices you make will help to renew activities or passions from your past or reinvent yourself along the lines of a new pursuit. Even if you feel satisfied with your current situation, there are always things you can do to further enrich your life and those of others around you. For someone in the ninth stage, you can generate new ideas for meaningful activities.

To begin the process of renewal or reinvention, I suggest that you take action based on the thinking and doing action verbs from the five types of wisdom that we develop as we age. I call these actions your *age imperatives*, and they are described on page 181.

The age imperative action plan stems directly from your wisdom chart and age culture, and lays out what you are doing now and what you could do in the future, either as a continuation of current activities, new activities, or contingency plans if you have anticipated limitations. Now take a sheet of paper and create your own age imperative action plan based on the template shown on page 182.

This grid is similar to Gene Cohen's "social portfolio," which consists of a personalized list of activities that one can do under two basic conditions: low or high mobility and individual or group pursuits. For example, swimming is an activity that requires high

Age Imperatives

SAVANT: LEARN and TEACH Ninth stage: OBSERVE and RECOLLECT	Select one ongoing educational activity that involves active, interactive learning or teaching. Examples: attend lifelong learning courses (learn); serve as school volunteer (teach). *Ninth stage examples:* Engage in active observing, such as listening to music, watching a ballet, or visiting a nature center (observe); talk about past memories (recollect).
SAGE: WEIGH and DECIDE Ninth stage: ATTEND and SUPPORT	Select some activity or involvement that involves discussion, debate, or involvement in decision making. Examples: participate in a book club (weigh); join a board of directors to help oversee an organization (decide). *Nine stage examples:* Be present at important events or ceremonies, such as a wedding, Sunday Mass, or Mother's/Father's Day brunch (attend) and have the opportunity to express interest and joy (support).
CURATOR: CARE and CONNECT Ninth stage: TEND and REPRESENT	Participate or volunteer for a group or organization in which you are supporting its cause, mission, or intergenerational interactions. Examples: attend political rallies (care); serve as a docent at a museum or a guide at a nature center (connect), *Ninth stage examples:* Participate in cultivation of plants or activities with animals (tend); participate in family, civic, or cultural events that honor or celebrate certain memories, values, or customs, such as holding an infant on your lap during a baptism or ritual circumcision, or carrying a flag during an Independence Day parade (represent).
CREATOR: IMAGINE and CREATE	Find an activity, hobby, or class in which you are making something new and different. Examples: act in a local theater (imagine); attend art classes (create). *Ninth stage examples:* Participate in creative storytelling (imagine) or guided painting or sculpting (create).
SEER: ACCEPT and COMMUNE Ninth stage: SANCTIFY	Get involved in a spiritual, religious, or intergenerational group or relationship in which there are customs, rituals, or communing together for a higher purpose. Examples: read from a religious book each day or listen to an inspirational religious leader (accept); attend a weekly religious service (commune). These also apply in the ninth stage, but certain events or rituals can be made even holier by the participation of an elder (sanctify).

Age Imperative Action Plan

AGE IMPERATIVES	What you do or can do now	What you can do in the future
Learn and Teach (Savant)		
Weigh and Decide (Sage)		
Care and Connect (Curator)		
Imagine and Create (Creator)		
Accept and Commune (Seer)		

Age Imperative Action Plan (Ninth Stage)

AGE IMPERATIVES	What they do or can do now	What they can do in the future
Observe and Recollect (Savant)		
Attend and Support (Sage)		
Tend and Represent (Curator)		
Imagine and Create (Creator)		
Accept, Commune, and Sanctify (Seer)		

mobility but can be done as an individual or in groups, whereas gardening can be accomplished with low mobility as an individual. Cohen proposes that a social portfolio be developed with the input of close family and friends, be as diversified as possible, and include activities as "insurance" that can be pursued even in the face of more severe physical or cognitive limitations. These principles apply as well to the age imperatives, and by deriving them from a broad wisdom chart and age culture, such considerations should already be built in.

It is important to include artistic pursuits in your age imperatives, especially for individuals in the ninth stage. My friend and colleague Elizabeth Lokon makes the point that "art is fundamental to being human, all the way back to preliterate societies who drew on cave walls."

Born in Jakarta, Indonesia, to an ethnically Chinese family, Lokon studied art and gerontology. In 2007, she founded a program at Miami University in Oxford, Ohio, to involve individuals with cognitive impairment in the visual arts, and called it Opening Minds through Art, or OMA. Lokon laments the fact that too many people reject artistic activities because they don't believe they have talent, but for her it's not about one's ability. "We all have a basic need for artistic expression," she explains. "It's a form of nourishment like water, food, and social relationships." In her work, she has seen how even individuals with severe cognitive limitations can blossom once they begin to express themselves artistically. Art distinguishes us from other animals; without it, we are less human, she believes.

Step 4: Legacy

Consider your legacy. My maternal great-grandparents Aaron and Belle had a single item on their bucket list, and that was to see the Holy Land. In 1925, they set out on a three-month journey from their home in a small Wisconsin town, first traveling by car and then train to New York Harbor. There, they boarded a ship to venture across the Atlantic Ocean and through the Mediterranean Sea, steaming along the coast of Italy and beneath the imposing cone of Mount Vesuvius, until finally gliding into Haifa Harbor under the gleaming eye of Mount Carmel. Aaron chronicled their pilgrimage across the nascent British mandate in a small notebook, writing about how they marveled at the budding agricultural colonies, sweated in the hot and dusty air, wept at the Tomb of Rachel, and prayed with fervor at the Western Wall.

Their trip was nothing like many of the bucket-list trips people take today, jetting off to mountain or island resorts to ski, snorkel, or simply lounge by the pool or beach with one hand on the photo button of a smartphone and the other cradling a piña colada. There were no gourmet meals, Ivy League lecturers, or expensive shopping excursions on their itinerary. Their trip was not about pleasure but about passion. They were on a mission that literally represented a bucket-list item across countless generations that they had the honor to finally fulfill. They journeyed as much for themselves as for their children and grandchildren, and these descendants are still influenced and inspired by this trip nearly ninety years later. I have seen similar pilgrimages, explorations, and excursions pursued by many aging friends and patients, including family trips back to Poland, China, Cuba, or Spain to trace one's roots; connect with something deeper; and pass along a sense of identity, values, and culture to one's family and friends. These are mindful quests with a ringing message that declares: "This is who we were, this is who we are, and this is who we shall be."

Aging enables us to fully appreciate and disseminate these messages about our identity and legacy. The task may be as immediate as being present at a family celebration or as complex as leading a trip back to one's ancestral home. It might be as simple as teaching a young family member to make a cherished recipe or sew a distinctive quilt, or as challenging as educating teenagers about one's traumatic experiences during wartime. Either way and in whatever form, we begin to understand that the fruits of our aging—the crown of wisdom and the whole gown and scepter of our existence—extends far beyond our own lifetime.

Consider two well-known acts of legacy. The first was David Bowie's award-winning music album *Blackstar*, released in 2016 just two days before his death at the age of sixty-nine from liver cancer. The second was Leonard Cohen's acclaimed *You Want It Darker*, released in 2016 just three weeks before his death at the age of eighty-two. Bowie's album is a mournful, mystical swan song, with lyrics alluding to his imminent death ("Look up here, I'm in Heaven") and imagery that caps the course of his creative life, such as the appearance in the video for the song "Blackstar" of a jewel-encrusted skull in a spacesuit reposing on an eerie distant planet, no doubt evoking the final resting place of Bowie's lost astronaut Major Tom from his 1969 song "Space Oddity." Cohen's album is a swansong with an equal focus on his impending death, and was produced in his own living room where he was confined due to severe pain. The lyrics of the titular song proclaim his awareness and acceptance of his fate: "Hineni, hineni ["I am here," in Hebrew], I'm ready, my lord."

These two remarkable works of art, rendered by individuals facing certain death, speak to the power of creating a legacy for others, defined as a gift or some other entity handed down from one generation to the next. The aging process enables us to see with optimal clarity the lives we've lived and the impact we've had. It forces reflection on the value and consequences of our decisions and creations. Even though we will not be present to see our full legacy, we can live a small part of it, and its pursuit can provide a powerful purpose in our lives as we try our best to craft its influence ahead of time.

For Bowie and Cohen, the impact of their music was and will continue to be profound. They were able to say what they wanted to say, knowing that millions of people will be listening for years to come. For others, legacy is less certain, and my Miami cabinet had strong thoughts on this topic. Sydell defined legacy broadly as

"Everything. Anything. Albums, pictures, tchotchkes. We try all our lives to tell the kids our feelings. Hopefully they can use what we gave them." Shirley was realistic about her limitations, telling the group that no matter how hard we work to establish an identity for our families and communities, it is not up to us but to the individuality of younger people to determine our true legacy. The group agreed. You try your best. You plan. In the end, there is no certainty, but it's still worth the effort.

Return now to the age culture grid and the fourth box, entitled "Legacy." Ask yourself what you want to leave behind for loved ones and for the future of your community, culture, or wider world. The answers may prompt important decisions or creative endeavors. In some ways, this legacy is a tenth stage of existence in which even in our passing we guarantee the renewal of meaning and hope. For some people, their legacy may consist of one or more preserved objects from the past that tell certain stories or history, such as an army uniform, a wedding dress, or a piece of sentimental jewelry. For others, it is a symbolic object that transmits one's culture or religion, such as an annotated book of recipes, a prayer book, or a family Bible. Legacy may also be transmitted through verbal or written stories, video messages, or statements of belief and instruction recorded in an ethical will.

For Peter, part of his legacy came through a dramatic appearance holding court at a large family reunion, where he was amazed by the attention he got from younger family members. His words became a legacy of sorts, and he was thrilled to share his perspectives. Peter reflected on his ninety years, starting as the seventh of eight children or "lucky number seven" to a Greek Orthodox family that traces its roots back to Sparta. His family gave him his grounding and his ethics, and good fortune has followed him ever since, he believes. He was a yeoman on the USS *Dempsey* destroyer escort during World War II, and on his return from the war helped to run his family business and then later got involved in the television industry. He married in 1962, was widowed in 1986, and then married again in 1989. He has two wonderful daughters who reflect the qualities of both his wives. Peter later reinvented himself as a real estate broker, took a big financial hit during the Wall Street crash of 2008, but picked himself up again. He told the group that the term *aging* should indicate more than decline and finality; it should signify a new beginning. That has been his experience even into his nineties. Although he doubts he'll live to 104 like his father, he is happy to listen to others and keep his own counsel, but is equally satisfied to tell his tales to those younger people who seek his wisdom.

Step 5: Celebration

Plan a ritual to celebrate your aging. We have rituals for every major transition in life, but almost none for aging. Anthropologist Barbara Myerhoff described how aside from retirement and funerals as the "crude markers for the stark beginning and end of old age," aging individuals are left facing multiple later life transitions without the benefit "of ritual, ceremony, or symbol." Even at the celebration of older birthdays, we do not herald aging itself as a positive and dynamic force. If anything, we do the opposite and denigrate aging with jokes, putdowns, and goofy cards that poke fun at our aches, pains, and failings. There are certainly many rituals of daily life in various cultures that are predominant domains of aged individuals, but few of these represent specific ways to honor late-life transitions or the aging process itself. Several clergy of various religious traditions have developed rudimentary ceremonies marking auspicious birthdays, but there are no mainstream approaches. There is a National Grandparents Day in the United States and fourteen other countries, but these celebrations are not widely observed. We are left with a blank slate.

We need ways to celebrate our aging self and the strengths we are gaining, and rituals and ceremonies can be important and powerful markers of this process. Think about what it means to you when you engage in such popular rituals as singing happy birthday to someone, wearing a cap and gown at a graduation ceremony, or toasting someone at a wedding. Such actions bring happiness and a sense or order, meaning and comfort. In their guidebook to creating late-life rituals called *Transitional Keys*, Andrea Sherman and Marsha Weiner describe how we can create new rituals to celebrate the value of aging individuals and symbolize their transition to higher degrees of wisdom and new roles in life. Such rituals also transmit the value of aging as a positive force to younger generations and the wider community. As a result, they provide support and meaning to those aging individuals who might otherwise feel cast aside.

Once you have completed reviewing your wisdom chart, age points, age culture, and age imperatives, consider holding a gathering or party to celebrate your aging self, using several rituals and ceremonies you create. Sherman and Weiner propose the following structure to such a celebration:

Beginning: Call the celebration to order and state its reason. The whole point here is to mark out a sacred time in which you will engage in meaningful and symbolic actions to celebrate the aging life of you or someone else. Consider a symbolic transition into the ceremony by passing through some form of designated threshold or entrance. The ritual space should be demarcated through sensory stimulation with meaningful music, decorations, costumes, hats, photographs, artwork, foods, scents, and symbolic objects.

A central table can hold treasured items that will be part of the celebration.

Middle: Have an activity to carry out the honoring and celebrating of the person. Several suggestions include:

- Talks and toasts about the strengths, lessons, wisdom, or other things that aging has brought you or the person you are honoring
- Display and discussion of symbolic objects representing your wisdom and purpose in life
- Presentation of symbolic, age-affirming gifts to the person being celebrated
- Presentation to attendees of symbolic gifts, writings, or messages from the person being honored
- Reading, chanting, or singing of relevant and meaningful prayers, poems, stories, or songs
- The composition of a special recipe, poem, reading, or song
- A special focus on the role of children and grandchildren to talk about or hear about the value of the person (e.g., a living eulogy)
- A ritual to symbolize growth and transition (e.g., wearing a ceremonial garment, such as a cap with embroidered colors or patterns to symbolize wisdom; exchanging an old symbolic object for a new one, such as turning over the car keys to symbolize the end of driving, but receiving a bowl with cards from everyone willing to offer rides)
- Involvement of relevant clergy, local officials, and/or official proclamations to recognize the importance and sacredness of the person or transition

Ending: Complete the ceremony with a closing that restates the purpose of the event and includes a call to the future and the legacy of the person.

These ideas can improve and ritualize a standard late-life birthday, or create a unique celebration unto itself. There is no accepted word to represent this celebration of aging, so I might suggest that you create your own meaningful term. For example, the southwestern Australian city of Warrnambool created the annual Celebrage Festival to encourage individuals older than sixty to get involved in new activities. It's not a ceremony per se, but it does promote a positive take on aging and has a great name. Savina Teubal created the Simchat Chochmah ceremony (Hebrew for "rejoicing in wisdom") for her sixtieth birthday as a ritual to celebrate her transition into later life. You might have terminology from a native language or from religious or cultural traditions that can help to name your own meaningful celebration.

Epilogue

IN 1947, TWO young men embarked on a gamble. The pair consisted of a medical student named Roy Walford and a mathematician named Albert Hibbs, and they headed into the casinos of Reno to test out a statistical model of roulette wheel performance that promised a cash windfall if their calculations proved correct. The gamble paid off handsomely, successfully parlaying their initial $300 investment into thousands of dollars, but eventually getting foiled by the wised-up croupiers and their overseers, who switched out the wheel. No bother—their winnings over time paid for school and a yacht to sail the Caribbean.

Years later, Dr. Roy Walford, then a distinguished professor of pathology at UCLA, embarked on a second gamble. Based on his studies with mice in which he discovered he could double their life span by feeding them 50 percent less food, Walford became both a proponent and a practitioner of caloric restriction as a way for himself and others to improve the quality and length of life. He wrote two best-selling books on life extension, and was one of the eight crew members who was sealed inside a huge terrarium called the Biosphere 2 between 1991 and 1993 to simulate how humans might live and sustain themselves in an enclosed ecosystem on other planets. Even as the Biosphere's plan to live completely and safely on homegrown food and recycled air was faltering, Walford proposed caloric restriction as a healthy strategy within the bubble.

Walford's gamble was that caloric restriction would improve and lengthen his life and that of other adherents, including his daughter Lisa. It's a gamble not unlike so many of the lifestyle choices that many people make every day hoping to have a longer, healthier life: rigorous exercise programs, megavitamin regimens, exotic herbal extractions, gluten-free diets, hormone injections and supplements, etc., etc. The list is long and each approach is ultimately a gamble based on variable science but little long-term data. Walford himself died from amyotrophic lateral sclerosis at the age of seventy-nine, uncertain of whether caloric restriction helped or hindered his life span. Regardless, his daughter Lisa spoke to me about the richness of his life as a true Renaissance man—doctor, scientist, activist, performer, writer, and filmmaker.

We don't know whether Walford's theory or any other strategy will someday make a significant difference in how long and how well we age. Nonetheless, we are already seeing the future of aging in front us through the lives of so-called superagers—individuals whose mind and body are extraordinarily bright and active well into their eighties, nineties, and beyond. Telltale signs of progress are emerging. For example, the average human life span is climbing to over eighty years in many countries, with centenarians being one of the fastest-growing single age groups. Death rates from cancer are declining and even the incidence of dementia has actually fallen in certain populations.

These trends will accelerate as we begin to cure more forms of cancer, find more effective ways to prevent and treat heart disease, reduce dementia risk factors, and eventually discover a cure for Alzheimer's disease. At that point, with the three greatest killers in check, the average person with access to good medical care and nutrition will have a hearty three to four decades of life beyond the typical age of retirement. What will such a life look like? We don't have to look further than ourself and all the other aging individuals around us! We have always had the tools to begin plotting our life in such a future.

CR

I began this book with the assertion that aging brings strengths, and I centered my arguments on three questions and their answers:

Why age? *To grow in wisdom.*
Why survive? *To realize a purpose.*
Why thrive? *To create something new.*

We all face these fundamental questions of aging, and the answers provide us with the potential to make aging what we want it to be, for ourself and for others who need our help when they are limited in their abilities. Nothing is guaranteed in later life and the challenges are many, but we must have hope. The best of research into longevity tells us that if we translate this hope into positive attitudes about aging and a sense of purpose, we not only live longer, but we live better. The essential Fountain of Youth formula that we have sought for centuries has been inside of us all along, but it is paradoxically not about seeking youth but about seeking age itself.

In the not-so-distant past, aging was venerated because it served an essential purpose in the family, tribe, or community. Its relative rarity conferred a mystique upon those aged individuals fortunate enough to survive the rigors of time. Their lives were seen as precious and indicative of divine reward, like the long-lived biblical figures whose lives and deeds reflected purity and purpose. Today, old age is neither venerated nor rare. We see the aging process in all its glory and destruction. Nothing is hidden and most people make it to late life, regardless of purity or purpose. Sadly, our view has become increasingly distorted by values that place independence, movement, and memory over everything else. We fear an aged life in which any of these factors falter, and we cast this version of old age as a villain. We aspire instead for an old age that is really youth in disguise, and spend billions on pills and potions and other treatments that promise to make us look and feel less old. In this illusion, the ultimate aphrodisiac of age is being able to fulfill one's bucket list without caring for a wider mission.

I have offered here an alternate view of aging as it is being experienced and celebrated by an increasing proportion of the population. As we age, we gain wisdom as a multifaceted form of mental currency that we store away year by year as a critical reserve, ready to yield its dividends. Our age-enhanced resilience gets us through adversity, proves our value to ourself and others, and enables us to discover our true purpose in life. We can respond to age-related changes by taking the best of our past and renewing it, or by letting go of certain parts and reinventing ourselves. These changes are led by our creative spirit, which grows and develops with age and enables us to realize a bursting, blooming age culture.

I argue that this alternate view of aging is as true and scientifically valid as Robert Arking's definition that I presented in the Introduction:

Aging is a time-dependent series of cumulative, progressive, intrinsic, and deleterious functional and structural changes that usually begin to manifest themselves at reproductive maturity and eventually culminate in death.

Given what we have learned, however, we can recast this definition of aging in a different but equally accurate manner:

Aging is an *experience*-dependent series of cumulative, progressive, intrinsic, and *positive psychological* changes that usually begin to manifest themselves at *midlife* and eventually culminate in *increased well-being.*

Aging gives us the brain power, abilities, connections, and resources to make this redefined notion of aging—and the experiences of our aging selves—as true as the standard definition based on decline and loss.

To age is the most profound thing we accomplish in life. It stitches together generations and enables the flow of culture and history. It allows us to fully appreciate the incredible power of our individual age cultures, and to understand how we are like the keystone species of an ecosystem, whose very presence enables health, stability, and growth. From this vantage point, we can begin again to venerate aging and the aged because of their essential roles in our family, community, and society. Ultimately, this message is a call to action for each one of us to begin shaping and reshaping aging in our own unique ways, guided and inspired by the lives of the most beloved, influential, and profound individuals who have gone before us.

As you age, then, number both the days and the details of your accomplishments. Wear your crown of wisdom with pride and never shy away from sharing it with those you care about. Measure yourself not by how you look but by how you rise. Hold tightly to the values and virtues of your past that define who you are, but do not be afraid to let go at times and step forward into a new light. Do not stand by when those too weakened by age, disability, or disease seem to fail at this task, but grab hold of them and help them shine as well. When we truly act our age, our strengths burst forth and allow us to create the life, love, and lasting legacy that truly make us the valuable and valued person we yearn to be. That is the end of being old and the beginning of aging with wisdom, purpose, and creativity.

Acknowledgments

IN MY ONGOING studies of the aging process, both in the clinic and in the pages of the many books that line my office, I have encountered hundreds of wonderful sayings and aphorisms. There is one that stands above them all in my mind because it speaks to the essence of my beliefs. It comes from Psalm 92: *Even in old age they will still produce fruit; they will remain vital and green.* The insight and the hopefulness of the psalmist who wrote this passage over twenty-five hundred years ago still amazes me, since the words were scribed at a time when old age was certainly rare and, when it did occur, quite rough. I offer my gratitude to this ancient, wise, and charitable soul who decided to inspire us toward what we could be as we aged, rather than to denigrate us for what we might become when illness, injury, and loss are at hand.

I offer my gratitude to many other similarly wise and charitable people who have inspired and supported the writing of this book. Let me begin by thanking my wife, Robin, and my three sons, Jacob, Max, and Sam, for their love and support along with their tireless interest in distracting me from writing to the more important tasks of living. I am blessed to have my parents, Ron and Belle Agronin, and my in-laws, Fred and Marlene Lippman, as supreme role models of aging. More than anyone else, they have shown me how aging brings strength. My parent's nonstop lives full of meaningful interests, pursuits, and relationships have amazed and inspired me and much of the material in this book. The same goes for my in-laws, who agreed to be featured in the chapter on age points.

My writing is directly inspired and supported by all my colleagues at Miami Jewish Health, where I have worked since 1999, and I am particularly grateful for the wonderful team that works with me in our memory and research center. I am fortunate to work with countless individuals on our beautiful campus in the heart of Miami who are dedicated to providing the very best of care for aging individuals in our community. We are working diligently to create the very first village setting in the United States for individuals with Alzheimer's disease and other forms of dementia, based on a model of care in which empathy is the guiding instinct.

I am thankful for the many friends, colleagues, patients, and caregivers who have allowed me to interview them or to share their stories, either in name or anonymously. They include, but are not limited to, Dr. Tanya Luhrmann, Rabbi Solomon Schiff, Archbishop Thomas Wenski, Imam Naseeb Khan, Lewis Richmond, John Preston, Leslee Geller, Dr. Dilip Jeste, Dr. Christopher Hertzog, Dr. Paul Verhaeghen, Victoria Haefner, Ruth Azaria, Hank Azaria, Sarah Rafferty, Dr. Elkhonon Goldberg, Irene Weisberg Zisblatt, Margarita Cano, Roslynn Averbook, Julie Newmar, Muriel Silverman, Ellyn Okrent, Dr. Carol Ryff, Bodi Lucas, Dr. Sarah Czaja, Liz Lerman, Katy Hessel, Dr. Patricia Jaegerman, Judy Lusskin, Shirley Falcone, Ken Jones, David Leddick, Peter Manners, Sydell Herrick, Alfred Herrick, Jim Banks, Norma Cox, Margaret Cox, Elizabeth Okon, Andrea Sherman, Lisa Walford, Bill Cherkasky, Rudy Cherkasky, and Dr. Alan Cherkasky. I offer thanks as well to Martin Ogawa and Andrew Hallenberg, who played key roles in promoting this book.

The book itself was inspired by Dr. Gene Cohen and has been supported by his life partner, Wendy Miller. Gabe Maletta was an invaluable mentor, friend, and colleague, and I would also like to dedicate its message to his memory. There are also several individuals who have supported my writing in important ways: Jane Gross, Charlie Wells, Jay Hershey, Demetria Gallegos, Cristina Lourosa, and Diane Ackerman.

This book itself would not exist without three specific individuals who have been my most stalwart supporters: my agent, Rafe Sagalyn; my editor, John Radziewicz; and my publicist, Lissa Warren. They understand both my passion and my mission as a geriatric psychiatrist and writer on the aging process. Working on a second book with this magnificent trio has been as satisfying as the first, and I cannot imagine either book without their guiding hands. I extend this gratitude to the entire team at Da Capo Press, Perseus Books Group, and Hachette Book Group who have worked diligently to review, edit, design, and promote this book.

ଓ

A few months before he died, my grandfather Dr. Simon Cherkasky insisted on buying me a gift for all the time I had spent talking to him while he was going through treatment for cancer. It had been an uncomfortable but necessary reversal—the young doctor fresh out of training now providing advice and care to the aged master clinician who also happened to be his own childhood doctor. I tried to imagine what item could possibly symbolize the connection I had with him, and after some thought I settled on a beautiful, old-fashioned leather briefcase that could double as a doctor's bag. I hoped that the briefcase would always remind me of my grandfather as I carried it into meetings and examinations with patients over the course of my career. Truth be told, most doctors, including myself, do not use doctor's bags anymore, and it now sits forlornly beneath my desk at home. It contains a treasure trove of old journal articles, pharmaceutical brochures, empty pillboxes, and an aging rubber reflex hammer, along with a layer of dust along its handsome rounded top and in the crevices of its handle and seams.

The bag is weighty and beautiful, but it's not my grandfather. It doesn't inspire my work like the moments I spent in my grandfather's presence. It doesn't help me to focus my eyes intently on a patient or lean forward and gesture with my hands in a reassuring manner the way I learned from my grandfather. As it ages, it seems more dusty and useless, nothing like the respect and awe I had for my grandfather as he aged. I am who I am not because of any object from my grandfather in my possession—the bag, his medical books and old stethoscopes, his *entire desk*—but because of the time I spent with him absorbing the knowledge, values, and character that he gained from aging. I am part of his essential legacy, as is all the good I've done as a doctor.

As much as I yearn for the elders from my past, I still have two amazing living consolations in the form of my great-uncles Bill and Rudy, younger brothers and physical avatars of my grandfather Simon. Bill is ninety-three years old, retired from his previous work in government, a World War II veteran and Bronze Star winner, an active golfer and regular e-mailer, and a patriarch for his family. Rudy is eighty-nine years old, retired from running the family dairy and bakery (with the best cream-filled donuts south of Green Bay!), an active skier, and, like his older brother, a regular e-mailer and the patriarch of his family. I am grateful to both my uncles for their advice and guidance with my thinking about aging for this book. They are stunning role models who truly exemplify the future of aging for all of us. They are wise, resilient, and creative. They are rooted in their lifelong values but are not afraid to make necessary changes to fit the situation. My family and I are blessed by their presence, and we all pray that we will be as sharp, sociable, and humorous as them as we age.

Notes

Epigraph

vii   **"Even if I could have done":** The quotation from Matisse appears in Hilary Spurling's *The Unknown Matisse: A Life of Henri Matisse: The Early Years, 1869–1908* (New York: Alfred A. Knopf, 1998), 29.

Introduction

2   **supercentenarian:** This refers to someone who has lived to or beyond the age of 110 years.

3   **lives of centenarians:** The best research on centenarians comes from the work of Thomas Perls. Some of his initial research is outlined in *Living to 100: Lessons in Living to Your Maximum Potential at Any Age* by Thomas T. Perls and Margery Hutter Silver (New York: Basic Books, 1999). A more recent article that summarizes his research is P. Sebastiani and T. T. Perls, "The Genetics of Extreme Longevity: Lessons from the New England Centenarian Study," *Frontiers in Genetics* 3 (2012): 277. In addition, the concept of "Blue Zones," where there are high average life spans, has been featured in Dan Buettner's *The Blue Zones: 9 Lessons for Living Longer (from the people who've lived the longest)*, 2nd ed. (Washington, DC: National Geographic, 2008/2012).

7   **In my previous book:** Marc E. Agronin, *How We Age: A Doctor's Journey into the Heart of Growing Old* (Cambridge, MA: Da Capo Press, 2011).

8   **"It's great to be old":** Susan Jacoby, *Never Say Die: The Myth and Marketing of the New Old Age* (New York: Pantheon Books, 2011).

9   **"living too long is also a loss":** Ezekiel Emanuel, "Why I Hope to Die at 75," *Atlantic*, October 2014, accessible at https://www.theatlantic.com/magazine/archive/2014/10/why-i-hope-to-die-at-75/379329/.

9   **"mindless, selfless, unreasonable creatures":** Kent Russell, "We Are Entering the Age of Alzheimer's," *New Republic*, September 2, 2014, accessible at https://newrepublic.com/article/119265/alzheimers-disease-statistics-show-illness-will-define-our-times.

10   **"Old age is the final act of life":** Marcus Tillius Cicero, "On Old Age," in *The Basic Works of Cicero*, ed. M. Hadas (New York: Random House, 1951 [44 BC]), 125–158. It is relatively easy to access the text of Cicero's essay through a simple Internet search.

10   **"The end of life is at hand":** From the writings of Ptah-Hotep as translated by Battiscombe G. Gunn in *The Instruction of Ptah-Hotep and the Instruction of Ke'Gemni: The Oldest Books in the World* (London: John Murray, 1906). The full text can be accessed online in "The Project Gutenberg Ebook," released November 20, 2009, at https://archive.org/stream/theinstructionof30508gut/pg30508.txt.

10   **life extension proponents:** Aubrey de Grey, with Michael Rae, *Ending Aging: The Rejuvenation Breakthroughs That Could Reverse Human Aging in Our Lifetime* (New York: St. Martin's Griffin, 2007); Ray Kurzweil and Terry Grossman, *Fantastic Voyage* (New York: Plume, 2005).

11   **a mechanistic series of steps:** Robert Arking's definition of aging can be found in *The Biology of Aging: Observations and Principles*, 3rd ed. (New York: Oxford University Press, 2006), 11.

Part I

17   **"An aged man is but a paltry thing":** From the poem "Sailing to Byzantium, by W. B. Yeats, in *The Tower* (New York: Scribner, 2004 [facsimile edition]). Originally published in 1928. The poem can be

accessed at https://www.poetryfoundation.org/poems-and-poets/
poems/detail/43291.

17 **"Old age allows us"**: Matis Weinberg, *FrameWorks: Bereishit/Genesis* (Boston: Foundation for Jewish Publications, 1999), 112–113.
With permission of the author.

Chapter 1

26 **"evil in all things"**: From the writings of Ptah-Hotep as translated
by Battiscombe G. Gunn in *The Instruction of Ptah-Hotep and the
Instruction of Ke'Gemni: The Oldest Books in the World* (London:
John Murray, 1906). The full text can be accessed online in "The
Project Gutenberg Ebook," released November 20, 2009, at https://
archive.org/stream/theinstructionof30508gut/pg30508.txt.

26 **"really bad for you"**: Aubrey de Grey, with Michael Rae, *Ending
Aging: The Rejuvenation Breakthroughs That Could Reverse Human
Aging in Our Lifetime* (New York: St. Martin's Griffin, 2007), 10.

26 ***theodicy,* or justification of evil:** Leibniz wrote about his thoughts
on why there is evil in a divinely created world in his 1709 work
Theodicy. A detailed description of his thinking can be found online
in the *Stanford Encyclopedia of Philosophy* at https://plato.stanford
.edu/entries/leibniz-evil/.

27 **evolutionary theory of aging:** A good review of this theory can be
found at http://www.senescence.info/evolution_of_aging.html.

28 **"Keepers of the Meaning" and "Guardians":** George E. Vaillant
writes about these concepts in his books *Aging Well* (Boston: Little,
Brown, 2002) and *Triumphs of Experience: The Men of the Harvard
Grant Study* (Cambridge, MA: Belknap Press, 2012).

28 **grandmother hypothesis:** There are many scientific articles on this
hypothesis, developed by anthropologist Kristen Hawkes and colleagues. Two good papers include: K. Hawkes, J. F. O'Connell, and
N. G. Blurton Jones, "Hadza Women's Time Allocation, Offspring
Provisioning, and the Evolution of Long Postmenopausal Life
Spans," *Current Anthropology* 38, no. 4 (1997): 551–557, accessible at:
https://collections.lib.utah.edu/details?id=702745; and K. Hawkes,
J. F. O'Connell, N. G. Blurton Jones, H. Alvarez, and E. L. Charnov,
"Grandmothering, Menopause, and the Evolution of Human Life

Histories," *Proceedings of the National Academy of Sciences of the United States of America* 95 (1998): 1336–1339, accessible at http://content.csbs.utah.edu/~hawkes/Hawkes_al98gramsHumanLife History%20PNAS.pdf. See also James G. Herndon's article "The Grandmother Effect: Implications for Studies on Aging and Cognition" in *Gerontology* 56, no. 1 (January 2010): 73–79, accessible at https://www.ncbi.nlm.nih.gov/pmc/articles/PMC2874731/.

29   **interesting tidbits and stories:** Solomon Schiff, *Under the Yarmulke: Tales of Faith, Fun, and Football* (Miami: Chai Books, 2011).

29   **legends from the Talmud:** From Louis Ginzberg, *Legends of the Bible* (New York: Simon & Schuster, 1956), 139.

30   **judge all people on the good side:** *Pirke Avot*, or *Sayings of Our Fathers*, is a traditional collection of Talmudic aphorisms. Rabbi Schiff was referring to a passage in the first chapter (1:6) that reads: "Yehoshua ben Perakhyah said provide yourself with a teacher, acquire for yourself a friend, and judge every person favorably."

31   **interreligious dialogue on faith:** Abraham Skorka, Marcelo Figueroa, and Jorge Mario Bergoglio [Pope Francis], *The Bible: Living Dialogue—Religious Faith in Modern Times* (Philadelphia: American Bible Society, 2015), 139.

31   **"forsook the counsel of the old men":** The passage is from Kings 12:8, quoted here from a translation by A. Cohen, *Soncino Books of the Bible: Kings* (London: Soncino Press, 1950), 92.

32   **dual perspectives in Buddhist thinking:** Lewis Richmond, *Aging as a Spiritual Practice: A Contemplative Guide to Growing Older and Wiser* (New York: Gotham Books, 2012).

33   **self-fulfilling prophecy:** One of the best advocates for developing a positive narrative of aging to counteract common ageist beliefs is age critic and theorist Margaret Morganroth Gullette, notably stated in her book *Agewise: Fighting the New Ageism in America* (Chicago: University of Chicago Press, 2011).

33   **"stereotype embodiment theory":** B. R. Levy, M. Slade, S. Kunkel, and S. Kasl, "Longevity Increased by Positive Self-perceptions of Aging," *Journal of Personality and Social Psychology* 83 (2002): 261–270.

33   **"counterclockwise study":** Ellen J. Langer, *Counterclockwise: Mindful Health and the Power of Possibility* (New York: Ballantine Books, 2009).

34   **Baltimore Longitudinal Study on Aging:** In this study, individuals aged eighteen to forty-nine were followed over thirty-eight years. For more information, go to http://www.blsa.nih.gov.

34   **significantly positive attitude toward aging:** Levy et al., "Longevity."

34   **Middle Age in the United States (MIDUS) Study:** A full description can be found at http://www.midus.wisc.edu.

34   **"socioemotional selectivity theory":** Laura L. Carstensen, *A Long Bright Future: An Action Plan for a Lifetime of Happiness, Health, and Financial Security* (New York: Broadway Books, 2009).

35   **eight stages of life:** Erik H. Erikson, *Childhood and Society* (New York: W. W. Norton, 1950).

36   **"Hope may easily give way to despair":** Erik H. Erikson and Joan M. Erikson, *The Life Cycle Completed* (New York: W. W. Norton, 1997), 107.

Chapter 2

41   **"A life honorably and virtuously led":** Marcus Tillius Cicero, "On Old Age," in *The Basic Works of Cicero*, ed. M. Hadas ((New York: Random House, 1951 [44 BC]), 125–158.

41   **I was the visiting psychiatrist:** The opening story is based upon (and borrows a few phrases from) a piece I wrote called "Sunshine," published in *CNS News* 9, no. 10 (October 2007): 24–25.

43   **experts on late-life schizophrenia:** D. V. Jeste, L. L. Symonds, M. J. Harris et al., "Non-dementia Nonpraecox Dementia Praecox? Late-Onset Schizophrenia," *American Journal of Geriatric Psychiatry* 5 (1997): 302–317.

44   **the sacred Hindu scripture of the Bhagavad Gita:** D. V. Jeste and I. V. Vahia, "Comparison of the Conceptualization of Wisdom in Ancient Indian Literature with Modern Views: Focus on the Bhagavad Gita," *Psychiatry* 71, no. 3 (2008): 197–209.

46   **our brain's abilities as we age:** Several excellent reviews on cognitive changes in late life include the following: B. W. Palmer and S. E. Dawes, "Cognitive Aging," in *Successful Cognitive and Emotional Aging*, ed. C. A. Depp and D. V. Jeste (Washington, DC: American Psychiatric Publishing, 2010), 37–54; P. Verhaeghen and

C. Hertzog, *The Oxford Handbook of Emotion, Social Cognition, and Problem Solving in Adulthood* (New York: Oxford University Press, 2014); and T. A. Salthouse, *Major Issues in Cognitive Aging* (New York: Oxford University Press, 2010).

47   **greater comprehension:** C. Jennifer, J. C. Weeks, and L. Hasher, "The Disruptive—and Beneficial—Effects of Distraction on Older Adults' Cognitive Performance," *Frontiers in Psychology* 5 (2014): 133.

49   **Berlin wisdom paradigm:** A good website that reviews Paul Baltes's model of wisdom is http://www.berlinwisdommodel.weebly.com.

51   **"honored by all, adorned with holy diadems":** This quote is taken from the surviving fragment of the Greek philosopher Empedocles's (490–430 BCE) poetic work *Purifications*.

51   *brain reserve*: A. M. Brickman, K. L. Siedlecki, and Y. Stern, "Cognitive and Brain Reserve," in *Successful Cognitive and Emotional Aging*, ed. C. A. Depp and D. V. Jeste (Washington, DC: American Psychiatric Publishing, 2010), 157–172.

52   **scaffolding theory of aging and cognition:** D. C. Park and P. Reuter-Lorenz, "The Adaptive Brain: Aging and Neurocognitive Scaffolding," *Annual Review of Psychology* 60, no. 1 (2009): 173–196.

52   **CRUNCH:** J. O. Goh and D. C. Park, "Neuroplasticity and Cognitive Aging: The Scaffolding Theory of Aging and Cognition," *Restorative Neurology and Neuroscience* 27 (2009): 391–403. Also see D. C. Park and P. Reuter-Lorenz, "Human Neuroscience and the Aging Mind: A New Look at Old Problems," *Journals of Gerontology, Series B, Psychological Sciences and Social Sciences* 65B, no. 4 (July 2010): 405–415.

52   **One study of elite pianists:** R. T. Krampe and K. A. Ericsson, "Maintaining Excellence: Deliberate Practice and Elite Performance in Young and Older Pianists," *Journal of Experimental Psychology General* 125, no. 4 (December 1996): 331–359.

52   **"superagers":** F. W. Sun, M. R. Stepanovic, J. Andreano, L. F. Barrett, A. Touroutoglou, and B. C. Dickerson, "Youthful Brains in Older Adults: Preserved Neuroanatomy in the Default Mode and Salience Networks Contribute to Youthful Memory in Superaging," *Journal of Neuroscience* 36, no. 37 (September 14, 2016): 9659–9668.

55   **expert at pattern recognition:** Elkhonon Goldberg, *The Wisdom Paradox* (New York: Gotham Books, 2006).

55   **aging cognition is better able to integrate and balance:** One of the best proponents of adult cognitive development is Gisela LaBouvie-Vief. See her 1982 paper "Growth and Aging in Life-span Perspective," *Human Development* 25, 65–78. Her work is based on what has been called postformal or dialectical thinking. These concepts are highlighted in R. A. Nemiroff and C. A. Colarusso, eds., *New Dimensions in Adult Development* (New York: Basco Books, 1990). In addition, Robert Sternberg's balance theory of wisdom is predicated on these changes in our cognition, as he believes that wisdom involves a necessary balancing of various interests, environments, and potential consequences in making decisions.

56   **the center for emotional regulation:** A wonderful explanation of these changes in aging brain function can be found in Louis Cozolino's *The Healthy Aging Brain: Sustaining Attachment, Attaining Wisdom* (New York: W. W. Norton, 2008).

59   **Irene wrote a book:** Irene Weisberg Zisblatt and Gail Ann Webb, *The Fifth Diamond* (Ithaca, NY: Ithaca Press, 2008).

60   **Vaillant's curator equivalents:** The best description of "guardians" can be found in George E. Vaillant, *Triumphs of Experience: The Men of the Harvard Grant Study* (Cambridge, MA: Belknap Press, 2012), 155.

60   **empathy and altruism:** One excellent article is J. N. Beadle, A. H. Sheehan, B. Dahlben, and A. H. Gutchess, "Aging, Empathy, and Prosociality," *Journals of Gerontology, Series B: Psychological Sciences and Social Sciences* 70, no. 2 (2015): 213–222. Another is Y. C. Chen, C. C. Chen, J. Decety, and Y. Cheng, "Aging Is Associated with Changes in the Neural Circuits Underlying Empathy," *Neurobiology of Aging*, 35, no. 4 (2014): 827–836.

62   **Margarita Cano:** Margarita's painting *¡Libertad!* can be viewed at http://www.floridadreaming.net/margarita-cano/. Her quote can be found at http://calendar.mdc.edu/EventList.aspx?view=Event Details&eventidn=14189&information_id=56739&type=& syndicate=syndicate. Her second quote is from an artist's statement and can be found at http://www.crematafineart.com/artists/ Cano/bio.html.

63   **the guru of creativity in late life:** See Gene Cohen's books *The Creative Age: Awakening Human Potential in the Second Half of Life* (New York: HarperCollins, 2000) and *The Mature Mind: The Positive Power of the Aging Brain* (New York: Basic Books, 2005).

63   *developmental intelligence:* Defined by Cohen in *The Mature Mind* as the "degree to which an individual has manifested his or her unique neurological, emotional, intellectual, and psychological capacities."

64   **motivational reserve:** See A. Maercker and S. Forstmeier, "Healthy Brain Ageing: The New Concept of Motivational Reserve," *Psychiatrist* 35 (2011): 175–177.

64   **Advanced Style:** Women that have been photographed as part of Advanced Style can be viewed at http://www.advanced.style.

65   **"I remember better when I paint":** For more on Hilgos and the documentary, go to http://www.irememberbetterwhenipaint .com. Berna Heubner's book is entitled *I Remember Better When I Paint: Art and Alzheimer's—Opening Doors, Making Connections* (Bethesda, MD: Bethesda Communications Group, 2012).

67   **seers channel their spiritual selves:** See Dan Blazer and Keith Meador's "The Role of Spirituality in Healthy Aging," in *Successful Cognitive and Emotional Aging*, ed. C. A. Depp and D. V. Jeste (Washington, DC: American Psychiatric Publishing, 2010), 73–86.

68   *gerotranscendence:* See Lars Tornstam's *Gerotranscendence: A Developmental Theory of Positive Aging* (New York: Springer Publishing, 2005).

Part II

73   **"When we talk about old age":** This quote is from Robert Butler's Pulitzer Prize–winning book *Why Survive?: Being Old in America* (New York: Harper & Row, 1975).

Chapter 3

88   **disengagement was a natural part of aging:** the *disengagement theory* of aging was first proposed by Elaine Cumming and William Earl Henry in their 1961 book *Growing Old* (New York: Basic Books) and stated that aging brought an expected process of disengagement from social connections. These changes, they

believed, were related to age-imposed losses of skills and roles that lessened an individual's previous social connections. There are two opposing theories: the *activity theory* states that individuals can optimize aging by engaging in social activities and interactions (described by R. J. Havighurst in his 1961 paper "Successful Ageing" in *Gerontologist* 1:8–13); the *continuity theory* proposes that individuals will tend to maintain previous pursuits and social connections as they age (described by R. C. Atchley in his 1989 paper "A Continuity Theory of Normal Aging," in *Gerontologist* 29, no. 2:183–190).

89 **"we will be diminished in one respect in order to grow in another":** From Marie de Hennezel's *The Art of Growing Old: Aging with Grace* (New York: Viking, 2012), 152–153.

Chapter 4

93 **impact of stress on the aging brain and body:** For a good discussion of the aging body's and brain's response to acute stress, I recommend Ruth O'Hara and colleagues' "Stress, Resilience, and the Aging Brain," in *Successful Cognitive and Emotional Aging*, ed. C. A. Depp and D. V. Jeste (Washington, DC: American Psychiatric Publishing, 2010), 173–196.

93 **In her account of the storm's fury:** See Ellis Anderson's *Under Surge Under Siege: The Odyssey of Bay St. Louis and Katrina* (Jackson: University Press of Mississippi, 2010).

94 **resilience:** See Steven Southwick and Dennis Charney's excellent resource *Resilience: The Science of Mastering Life's Greatest Challenges* (Cambridge, UK: Cambridge University Press, 2012).

94 **post-traumatic stress disorder (PTSD):** Ibid., 215–217.

94 **PTSD, aging is a neutral factor:** See Y. Barak, "Posttraumatic Stress Disorder in Late Life," in *Principles and Practice of Geriatric Psychiatry*, 2nd ed., ed. M. E. Agronin and G. J. Maletta (Philadelphia: Lippincott Williams & Wilkins, 2011), 515–522.

94 **study of older survivors of Hurricane Katrina:** S. Hrostowski and T. Rehner, "Five Years Later: Resiliency Among Older Adult Survivors of Hurricane Katrina," *Journal of Gerontological Social Work* 55, no. 4 (2012): 337–351.

99   **narrative and perhaps even an ideology of decline:** As noted in the notes for Chapter 1, see Margaret Morganroth Gullette's *Agewise: Fighting the New Ageism in America* (Chicago: University of Chicago Press, 2011).

100 **Erik Erikson's eighth stage of development:** Erik H. Erikson and Joan M. Erikson, *The Life Cycle Completed* (New York: W. W. Norton, 1997), 107. I would also recommend Erik H. Erikson, Joan M. Erikson, and Helen Q. Kivnick's book *Vital Involvement in Old Age* (New York: W. W. Norton, 1986).

100 **Grant Study of Adult Development:** See George E. Vaillant's books *Aging Well* (Boston: Little, Brown, 2002) and *Triumphs of Experience: The Men of the Harvard Grant Study* (Cambridge, MA: Belknap Press, 2012).

100 **Eight-Decade Study:** See Howard Friedman and Leslie Martin's *The Longevity Project: Surprising Discoveries for Health and Long Life from the Landmark Eight-Decade Study* (New York: Plume, 2012).

102 **Carol's work over the past three decades:** Dr. Carol Ryff has been a professor in the Department of Psychology at the University of Wisconsin in Madison for the past thirty years, where she is also the director of the Institute on Aging. She is also the director of the Midlife in the United States (MIDUS) study, which is a national longitudinal study of health and well-being. To read more about her model of well-being, consider the following three papers: C. D. Ryff, A. S. Heller, S. M. Schaefer, C. van Reekum, and R. J. Davidson, "Purposeful Engagement, Healthy Aging, and the Brain," in *Current Behavioral Neuroscience Reports*, published online October 22, 2016; C. D. Ryff and B. H. Singer, "Best News Yet on the Six-Factor Model of Well-being," *Social Science Research* 35 (2006): 1103–1119; and C. D. Ryff and B. H. Singer, "Know Thyself and Become What You Are: A Eudaimonic Approach to Psychological Well-being," *Journal of Happiness Studies* 9 (2008): 13–39.

106 **"say what we want to say":** Paraphrase of Matisse's comment: "Only what I created after the illness constitutes my real self: free, liberated. . . . I have needed all that time to reach the stage where I can say what I want to say." This quote and other details of Matisse's creativity in late life can be found at http://www.henri-matisse.net/

cut_outs.html and at http://www.luxebeatmag.com/henri-matisse
-cut-outs-tate-modern/.

106 **aging brings less stress and greater well-being:** One notewor-
thy survey is from A. A. Stone, J. E. Schwartz, J. E. Broderick, and
A. Deaton, "A Snapshot of the Age Distribution of Psychological
Well-being in the United States," *Proceedings of the Academy of
National Sciences* 107, no. 22 (2010): 9985–9990.

Part III

111 **"Aging and creativity":** Quote by Gene Cohen in *The Creative Age.
Awakening Human Potential in the Second Half of Life* (New York:
HarperCollins, 2000), 66.

Chapter 5

115 **"youthist":** This is a slang term defined in the Urban Dictionary as
"a being who contains large amounts of youth, pride, humor, and
justice. Who enjoys being who they are, what they do, and how they
do it. Who is not afraid of opinions. Who is charismatic and joyful"
(http://www.urbandictionary.com/define.php?term=Youthist).
This definition of *youth* equates being young with vitality, authenticity, and happiness, as if aging lacks those factors. The term is also
well represented by the website http://www.youthist.com, which
promotes antiaging products and strategies for "ageless" skin.

120 **a nostalgic point of view can counteract loneliness:** See W. Y.
Cheung, T. Wildschut, C. Sedikides, E. G. Hepper, J. Arndt, and
A. J. Vingerhoets, "Back to the Future: Nostalgia Increases Opti-
mism," *Personality and Social Psychology Bulletin* 39, no. 11 (2013):
1484–1496; and W. A. van Tilburg, E. R. Igou, and C. Sedikides, "In
Search of Meaningfulness: Nostalgia as an Antidote to Boredom,"
Emotion 13, no. 3:450–461. An interesting essay called "Nostalgia and
Its Discontents," based on Svetlana Boym's *The Future of Nostalgia*
(New York: Basic Books, 2001), can be found at https://pdfs.semantic
scholar.org/cfcb/eba8cb80315ffebfcf16fe4d17fa6f31286e.pdf.

120 **C. S. Lewis captured the risk of this pursuit:** The quote is from
an essay by noted British author C. S. Lewis entitled "The Weight

of Glory," first published in 1941. It can be accessed at http://www
.verber.com/mark/xian/weight-of-glory.pdf (page 3).

Chapter 6

131 **"There are no ordinary people"**: C. S. Lewis essay "The Weight
of Glory," first published in 1941, accessible at http://www.verber
.com/mark/xian/weight-of-glory.pdf (page 6).

131 **"good enough parent"**: This concept is described by D. W. Winnicott in *The Child, the Family, and the Outside World* (New York:
Penguin, 1973).

131 **"successful aging"**: The term has been used in many contexts, but
here I am referring to its description in John W. Rowe and Robert
L. Kahn's *Successful Aging: The MacArthur Foundation Study* (New
York: Pantheon Books, 1998).

132 **"positive aging"**: See Robert D. Hill's *Positive Aging: A Guide for
Mental Health Professionals and Consumers* (New York: W. W. Norton, 2005).

132 **SOC model of aging:** See P. B. Baltes and M. M. Baltes, "Psychological Perspectives on Successful Aging: The Model of Selective
Optimization with Compensation," in *Successful Aging: Perspectives from the Behavioral Sciences* (Cambridge, UK: Cambridge
University Press, 1990), 1–34.

133 *creative aging:* Gene Cohen's work can be found in his two books
*The Creative Age: Awakening Human Potential in the Second Half
of Life* (New York: HarperCollins, 2000) and *The Mature Mind:
The Positive Power of the Aging Brain* (New York: Basic Books,
2005). An excellent biography of Gene can be found in W. Andrew
Achenbaum's article "Gene D. Cohen, MD, PhD: Creative Gero-
Psychiatrist and Visionary Public Intellectual," *Journal of Aging,
Humanities, and the Arts* 4 (2010): 238–250.

134 **"Instead of what others warned"**: Cohen, *The Creative Age*, 126.

134 **"the secret of living with one's entire being" and "It can occur at
any age"**: Ibid., 17.

135 **the Paris fashion runways were bursting with color:** Katy Hessel's
excellent blog describes the impact that Matisse's cutouts had on
the Paris runways in 2014. It can be accessed at http://www.fashion
editoratlarge.com/tag/katy-hessel/.

136   **Henri Matisse:** The material on Matisse was largely based on three books: Hilary Spurling's monumental biographies *The Unknown Matisse: A Life of Henri Matisse—The Early Years, 1869–1908* (New York: Alfred A. Knopf, 1998); *Matisse the Master: A Life of Henri Matisse, The Conquest of Color, 1909–1954* (New York: Alfred A. Knopf, 2005); and Olivier Berggruen and Max Hollein, eds., *Henri Matisse: Drawing with Scissors—Masterpieces from the Late Years* (Munich: Prestel Berlag, 2006).

136   **"It's like being given a second life":** Spurling, *Matisse the Master*, 402.

136   **"From the moment I held the box of colours"** and **"Like an animal":** Spurling, *The Unknown Matisse*, 46

137   **"over the crack of old age"** and **"boisterous jokes":** Spurling, *Matisse the Master*, 415.

137   **"Even if I could have done":** Spurling, *The Unknown Matisse*, 29.

138   **"I have needed all that time":** This quote by Matisse can be found at http://www.henri-matisse.net/cut_outs.html.

138   **"It is the whole of me":** Spurling, *The Unknown Matisse*, 29.

138   **"there comes a time when a work has to be retired":** Martha Graham is quoted in Nan Robertson's article "Martha Graham Dances with the Future," *New York Times*, October 2, 1988, accessible at http://www.nytimes.com/1988/10/02/arts/martha-graham-dances -with-the-future.html?pagewanted=all.

139   **"our consumption is worth our contribution":** Ezekiel Emanuel, "Why I Hope to Die at 75," *Atlantic*, October 2014, accessible at https://www.theatlantic.com/magazine/archive/2014/10/why-i -hope-to-die-at-75/379329/.

139   ***The Eyes of the Goddess:*** The dance performance was reviewed by Anna Kisselgoff in "'Eyes of the Goddess,' a Fragment Left by Graham," *New York Times*, October 10, 1991, accessible at http:// www.nytimes.com/1991/10/10/arts/review-dance-eyes-of-the -goddess-a-fragment-left-by-graham.html.

140   **"Then one morning, I felt something welling up within me":** Martha Graham's recovery was detailed in her autobiography, *Blood Memory* (New York: Doubleday, 1991), 237.

141   **"It is the now that I must face and want to face":** Ibid., 276.

143   **this consummate creative choreographer has reinvented herself:** For her views on creativity, see Liz Lerman's *Hiking the Horizontal:*

Field Notes from a Choreographer (Middleton, CT: Wesleyan University Press, 2011).

144   **"human potential phases":** These phases are outlined in Gene Cohen's *The Mature Mind: The Positive Power of the Aging Brain* (New York: Basic Books, 2005).

148   **Henry A. Murray:** Henry Murray's writing can be found in *Endeavors in Psychology, Selections from the Personology of Henry A. Murray*, ed. Edwin S. Shneider (New York: Harper & Row, 1981). Forrest G. Robinson wrote a biography of Henry Murray called *Love's Story Told, A Life of Henry A. Murray* (Cambridge, MA: Harvard University Press, 1992). My own recollections of visiting with Murray also appear in a guest editorial entitled "Personality Is as Personality Does," *American Journal of Geriatric Psychiatry* 15, no. 9 (2007): 729–733.

149   **bronze medallion:** The design and origins of the medallion that bore the coat of arms for the Harvard Psychological Clinic can be found at: http://web.utk.edu/~wmorgan/tat/medall.htm.

149   **"full Congress of orators":** The quote is from H. E. Murray, "What Should Psychologists Do About Psychoanalysis?" *Journal of Abnormal and Social Psychology* 35 (1940): 50–175 (the quote appears on pages 160–161).

154   **"A bell with a crack":** From Diane Ackerman's *One Hundred Names for Love: A Stroke, a Marriage, and the Language of Healing* (New York: W. W. Norton, 2011), 302.

Part IV

157   **"I have needed all that time":** This quote by Matisse can be found at http://www.henri-matisse.net/cut_outs.html.

Chapter 7

178   **see ourself as actively growing with age:** Margaret Morganroth Gullette, *Agewise: Fighting the New Ageism in America* (Chicago: University of Chicago Press, 2011).

178   **"vital and free . . . constantly alternating between risk and success":** Described in Margret Stuffmann, "Jazz: Rhythm and Meaning," in *Henri Matisse: Drawing with Scissors—Masterpieces from*

the Late Years, ed. Olivier Berggruen and Max Hollein (Munich: Prestel Berlag, 2006), 24.

180 **"social portfolio":** Described in Gene Cohen's *The Mature Mind: The Positive Power of the Aging Brain* (New York: Basic Books, 2005).

187 **rituals for every major transition in life:** B. Myerhoff, "Experience at the Threshold: The Interplay of Aging and Ritual," in *Remembered Lives. The Work of Ritual, Storytelling, and Growing Older*, ed. Mark Kaminsky (Ann Arbor: University of Michigan Press, 1992). I strongly recommend reading Barbara Myerhoff's amazing book *Number Our Days* (New York: Simon & Schuster, 1978). The book was also made into an Academy Award–winning documentary of the same name.

188 **guidebook to creating late-life rituals:** Andrea Sherman and Marsha Weiner, *Transitional Keys. A Guidebook: Rituals to Improve Quality of Life for Older Adults* (New York: Transitional Keys, 2004). Read more at http://www.TransitionalKeys.org.

Epilogue

191 **two young men embarked on a gamble:** For an account of Roy Walford's adventures, see his obituary at http://www.articles.latimes.com/2004/may/01/local/me-walford1/2. A more detailed and interesting account can be found in Russell T. Barnhart's *Beating the Wheel: The System That Has Won over Six Million Dollars* (New York: Lyle Stuart, 1992).

191 **caloric restriction:** See Roy Walford's *Maximum Life Span* (New York: Avon, 1984) and *The 120 Year Diet* (New York: Simon & Schuster, 1986).

Index